ALLI SPOTTS-DE LAZZER
M.A., MFT, LPCC, CEDS

MEANING
FULL

23 LIFE-CHANGING STORIES OF CONQUERING DIETING, WEIGHT, & BODY IMAGE ISSUES

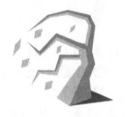

Unsolicited Press
Portland, Oregon
www.unsolicitedpress.com
orders@unsolicitedpress.com
619-354-8005

Cover Design: Kathryn Gerhardt
Editor: S.R. Stewart

ALLI SPOTTS-DE LAZZER
M.A., MFT, LPCC, CEDS

MEANING
FULL

23 LIFE-CHANGING STORIES OF CONQUERING DIETING, WEIGHT, & BODY IMAGE ISSUES

THE FINE PRINT

Medical/Mental Health: Nothing in this book should be considered a substitute for professional therapy or medical guidance. It's your responsibility to seek professional help.

Non-therapeutic Relationship: Reading of this book does not establish a therapeutic relationship between the reader and the author.

Recollection Accuracy: These are true-life stories, to the best of recollection. Memories can be subjective. Experiences have may been condensed, and selected dialogue may have been recreated, neither affecting the heart of the story.

Privacy: Some names and identifying details (those that are not vital to the stories) have been changed or combined to protect the privacy of individuals.

Non-endorsement: Any trademarks, service marks, or copyrights mentioned in this book are the property of their respective owners and do not indicate any endorsement or sponsorship. Also, unless stated, our Storytellers are not representing any brand and are sharing their own experiences.

Information Accuracy: Throughout time, information on health may evolve and change.

Disclaimer of Liability: Although the author and publisher have made every effort to ensure that the information in this book was correct at press time, the author and publisher do not assume and hereby disclaim any liability to any party for any loss, damage, or disruption caused by errors or omissions, whether such errors or omissions result from negligence, accident, or any other cause.

TABLE OF CONTENTS

INTRODUCTION

Don't eat this food; eat that food. Don't give up; work harder. Avoid this; add that. Good food; bad food. Good fat; bad fat. Good weight; bad weight. Healthy; not healthy. Do. Don't. Do. Don't.

Been there, done that? Are you ready for honest, uncomplicated, and doable solutions to your food, weight, and body image struggles? If you want to experience more contentment in life and to triumph over your eating and body battles, then read on.

As a Marriage and Family Therapist and specialist in eating and body image issues, I've been teaming with people to resolve their dieting, weight, and body image problems for over a decade. Previously, and like many of us, I also spent years struggling with dieting, healthy eating, and pushing my body to make it look different. I know that this helpful, motivational guide has been long overdue.

Both my personal and professional experience shape the content of *MeaningFULL: 23 Life-Changing Stories of Conquering Dieting, Weight, & Body Image Issues.* In these pages, you'll find relatable, honest, and inspiring stories of people who found keys to conquering:

- "failed" dieting;

- binge eating;

- emotional eating;

- unhealthy/healthy food choices;

- body dissatisfaction and body hate;

- yo-yo dieting (weight cycling);

- eating disorders; and

- related challenges (e.g., stressing about exercising, clean eating, or muscling up).

Each contributor shares the realizations and paths they followed that changed their food, dieting, weight, and body image problems into life-enhancing perspectives, practices, and skills. I'm pleased to offer you their discoveries, insights, and *hope*.

Following each narrative and major section in the book, I've inserted a "Note from Alli." The therapist in me wants you to have an additional view, a clarification, a useful exercise, or the science behind something discussed. For topics you may want to explore beyond these stories, I've provided supplemental, easily accessible online articles. My commentaries are intended to support you and broaden your options as you consider your path to finally conquering your issues.

Aware that eating and body image problems exist on a wide spectrum (from slight food and body-related frustrations to severe clinical eating disorders), I've made sure to include several stories about what's usually considered the most extreme—eating disorder recovery. Here's why: if someone's methods helped them to overcome a *serious* disorder, imagine how those methods might help you to overcome *your* issues, wherever they fall in the range from mild to intense.

Think of this book as visiting a store where everything in it relates to triumphing over dieting, weight, and body image issues. Each chapter is like an aisle that's both dedicated to your shopping experience and filled with relevant items. You get to pick and try out whatever interests you and leave anything on the shelf that doesn't.

As you read, you'll probably recognize parts of yourself in someone else's circumstances. You'll know that you're not alone in trying to manage (or master) these issues.

Each person's journey, solutions, and salvation are unique. Yours will be too. Through these diverse short stories, you'll discover useful ways to live a more fulfilled life—one freer from food, weight, and body image stresses and with improved wellness, too.

How the Heck Did We Get Here?

When we're babies and young children, we typically eat when we're hungry, stop eating when we're full, and let our bellies happily hang out with ever breath we take. For many of us, as we age, this natural connection with food and body gets distorted for various reasons. Consequently, terms that describe "disordered" relationships with eating and body are numerous: yo-yo dieting, binge eating, emotional eating, food obsession, body dissatisfaction, and more. Healthy lifestyle plans, weight-loss programs, and specific diets aimed at improving our relationship with food, weight, and body number even more so. (Which titles and brands quickly come to mind? The Paleo Diet, Keto Diet, Weight Watchers, intermittent fasting, Atkins Diet, HCG Diet, low-carb diet, low-fat diet...) Yet there are often unexpected, undesired byproducts of engaging in these remedies.

When we eat by following someone else's plan for how we "should" eat, we can diminish or lose our innate, internal connection with cravings, hunger, and fullness. That disconnection often leads people into tormenting food patterns and can bleed into questioning other areas of life too. *If I can't trust myself about when I'm hungry, what I crave, or if I'm full, how can I trust the rest of my internal guidance system? My gut-instinct? My decisions? My emotions? And so on.* Doubting one's internal guidance system tends to result in confusion, insecurity, missed opportunities, a lack of trust in self, unreliable decisions, and unwanted consequences; these then affect our relationships to our safety.

Even ordinary events frequently get complicated when we approach eating in manipulated ways. Think about the last time you attended a party while on a diet. Instead of focusing on the festivities and social interactions, you probably thought about the food (what you could/couldn't eat, the calories, the tastes, the food that others were consuming), right? In place of eating from automatic hunger and fullness cues that don't take much thought, our food rules require effort to maintain. In turn, this distracts us and tends to drain our energy.

Nevertheless, weight-loss plans, extreme healthy food practices, intense exercise regimens, and fad diets seem a *normal way of life* nowadays. In the media and social interactions, dieting, food, health, and body are common and constant topics of conversation. I invite you to do an experiment to test this: while in a public setting, take a few minutes to look at the visual messages surrounding you and to listen to others' conversations and on-air advertisements.

According to Marketdata LLC, there were 97 million active dieters[1] in America in 2016 (just under 1/3 of the country's entire population), and the U.S. weight-loss market worth had exceeded $72 billion[2] by 2019. Your body, weight, and attitudes about food and fat are (embrace the pun) big business. The pressure to fall in a specific range for body mass index (BMI, meaning weight to height ratio), coupled with the existing War on Obesity can cause even the wisest person to buy into a one-size-fits-all mentality.

---

[1] Marketdata LLC, *The U.S. Weight Loss & Diet Control Market*, (2017).
[2] Marketdata LLC. *The U.S. Weight Loss & Diet Control Market*, (2019).

There's an interesting video on YouTube by the Association of Size Diversity and Health called "The Problem with Poodle Science."[3] The short film brings to light that under the umbrella term "dogs," different breeds with naturally distinct physiques and requirements for health exist. It makes logical sense that a bullmastiff that loses enough pounds to weigh the same as a poodle is not a fit bullmastiff; it's a starved bullmastiff. Not everyone is supposed to be in a poodle's weight range, especially if you're a Chihuahua or a Great Dane. However, that's far from the message that permeates Western society.

We're constantly told (sometimes starting shortly after birth) that we need to change our bodies, sizes, shapes, weight, food intake, BMIs, etc. It's no wonder that so many of us feel desperate to accomplish these tasks.

What You're Going to Read

In these pages, you'll read concepts that may challenge what you believe to be the ultimate truth about weight, eating, or body image. An important reality is this: scientific, medical, mental health, and cultural paradigms about what's best and healthiest for us continue to evolve. So our own truths continue to evolve as well.

At this point, there are many philosophies and treatments geared towards stopping binge eating and emotional eating, increasing body acceptance, "winning the

---

[3] Herskowitz and Burgard, *The Problem with Poodle Science*, (2015).

battle" with weight or dieting, and the list goes on. None have been proven to be unequivocally *the way*. Additionally, conventional approaches may not yet offer *your* solutions for overcoming your food and body issues. Case in point: for some people, traditional dieting, even in the pursuit of health, can result in becoming unhealthy. (Confusing, right?) This will be clarified later in multiple chapters.

The following narratives came from contributors, also referred to as Storytellers, who voluntarily provided written drafts or recorded interviews. No one was paid to share their experience. As the curator, I worked with each inspiring Storyteller through the process, and each person's heart and journey moved me. In the pages that follow, you too will experience firsthand the incredible amount of support, passion, community, and creative problem-solving that's out there.

- This book has three main sections that follow my mini-memoir: "Discoveries," "Insights," and "Connections."

- In "Discoveries," the stories answer, *"How _____ is different now that I don't struggle with my food, weight, and body image issues."*

- In the second section, "Insights," our Storytellers share, *"What I wish I had known about _____ during my food, weight, and body image issues."*

- Section three, "Connections," contains narratives from family, friends, and teachers of people experiencing food and body stresses who answer, *"How _____ is different now that someone I care about seems freer from their food, weight, and body image issues."*

In each section, the narratives are brief and focused on hope. You will not be dragged through *all* the pain. Instead, I've aimed to offer just enough to appreciate the value in the shifts, the whys, and how-tos that can serve you.

Unless it's important to the journey, specific weight or size references have been omitted. This is because *what helps* often applies to a person of any size from *fat* through *skinny*. (If you just had an internal response to either italicized term, please give yourself a compassionate break. Try to see these words as straightforward dictionary definitions instead of loaded with self-criticism, merits, or judgments.)

Many experiences you'll read about don't contain a single "aha" or rock bottom moment that kicked someone into sudden change. Why? Because change often occurs through an ongoing and active process, piece-by-piece, and day-by-day. Gradually gaining insight or getting sick of repetition can propel a person towards movement. Many things can.

You're Not Alone

I recognize that if you're engaged in any level of struggle with your food or body, it may feel difficult to believe that a different life exists—one completely without (or at least with fewer) food-body-weight obstacles. Rest assured; there are many people out there who once felt similarly and no longer do.

Eating, weight, and body image problems can affect *anyone* of any size, gender, race, cultural identity, sexual orientation, financial status, religion, you name it. Though we are each diverse, we're connected like individual droplets of water that make up the ocean. You're not alone in your worries, failings, revelations, and triumphs.

For all of us, I think that finding our personal, potentially unorthodox keys to conquering these issues brings about change that makes life more meaningful.

Note from Alli:

For anyone who might feel skeptical about this book, I understand—years ago, I would have, too. You'll probably appreciate knowing that some Storytellers opted to remain anonymous or be given a pseudonym for the following reasons: uncertainty about the future of the Mental Health Parity Act (protection for pre-existing conditions), membership in a vulnerable population in the current political climate, or identity protection of those involved. For these Storytellers, identifying information within their narratives may have been altered. Their pertinent life stories remain intact. Also, you might notice that quite a few narratives mention a therapist who happens to be an eating disorders specialist; none refer to me.

As you read, please keep the following in mind. Each helps to clarify story content or to offer you personal safety measures.

- When eating issues are happening, even a mention of something related to food, size, or exercise can be upsetting. Also, some narratives contain raw and intense material. **Should you feel triggered (activated) by details anywhere in these pages,** please find someone to talk with, preferably a professional with experience in disordered eating or eating disorders.

- Various stories include adult content (e.g., strong language).

- Where appropriate, the gender-neutral pronouns "they/them/their" have been used to respect all genders.

- A unified understanding of clinical concepts and terms can help make a story more understandable and meaningful. If this could benefit you, please visit Concepts and Clarified Terms.

And now, get ready for a jarring, rebellious, inspiring book about conquering dieting, weight, and body image issues. It can change your life.

PROLOGUE

Alli's Clumsy Conquering—

My Story Leading to this Book

WHILE SEATED AT a dinner table for ten, people passed the last few bites of birthday cake around the table. With intense focus, I watched the plate move like a Ping-Pong ball at play. Some smiled and chatted as they tasted; others made irritating "mmmm" sounds. The pressure built amid the overly polite, drawn-out volley of discussion: "You have the last bite," "No, you have the last bite," "No, I simply couldn't!"

I snapped. My hand flew out across the table to stop the passing of the plate mid-Pong. I wish it had only been my thoughts, but I heard my voice rising over the volume of the noisy restaurant. Slowly and with precise enunciation, I boomed, "Fucking eat it, or don't eat it. But shut-up about it."

Heads turned. Abrupt silence fell across the table. All movement froze. Unusually wide eyes stared back at me. Blank faces. Jaws slightly dropped.

Shit.

I'd just ruined my best friend's 30th birthday.

While they'd been sharing stories about themselves, exchanging witty comments, and cracking each other up, I'd been growing increasingly agitated. By the time we reached dessert, I'd already endured two hours of my head unrelentingly screeching at me about all the food rules I'd broken.

I'd been feeling frustrated and ashamed of how challenging that dinner had been from its start to this finale. I also felt sad and selfish that I couldn't seem to pay attention to my friend like she deserved. I knew my window was closing for when I could get rid of what I'd eaten. My public happy mask slid off without my permission. I had lost control.

Since I usually smiled my way through discomfort, people rarely knew how much angst was going on in my head. That night, people saw it: the unease around food that had been visiting me, in varying intensities, since around 11 years old.

I'd already been on various diets before I hit my late tweens, when suddenly and without my consent or knowledge, my common dieting slipped into disorder, anorexia nervosa. Seemingly overnight, my favorite foods became inedible. Swallowing nearly anything other than my safe, steamed broccoli felt like a sandpaper-worm crawling down my throat. Obviously, this made eating a challenge.

Alarmed by my dramatic physical changes, like protruding vertebrae, my parents sought professional help. However, treatment in the 1980s was in its early stages. It was a terrible experience (super blaming on others) and caused me to mention little-to-nothing about food or weight in future therapy experiences.

After I gained enough pounds, I wasn't considered "anorexic" anymore. People seemed to think I was fixed and fine because I no longer looked sick.

I then spent decades on various regimens. Mostly, I tried to eat a "healthy" and low/no-fat diet and worked out for hours in the gym. I also replaced real foods with engineered food-like products. (As I write this, I can still taste my cinnamon toast made with saccharin and fake butter spray. Nasty.) I did the newest popular diets and followed celebrity diet-tips. One fad program I purchased had these weird pills that creepily filled your stomach once inside you. I mastered counting calories in and exercised off. I tried aids like over-the-counter diet pills that curbed my appetite but messed me up—they made me chase my speeding thoughts but not catch them. I smoked cigarettes to avoid eating. And I purged (got food inside me, out).

For years, I nonchalantly called these health and weight management practices my "maintenance." I accepted my demanding relationship with food and body as status quo. In public, people often complimented me on what they viewed as my "healthy choices" and "discipline." In private, the few who knew of the periods of bingeing and purging said little to nothing about it. One best friend used to stand in the bathroom doorway, chatting with me as she watched me make myself throw up. So, no big deal, right? Besides, I wasn't taking Fen-Phen, which I thought was way too severe and scary. I judgmentally elevated myself above anyone who did *that*. (Back then, everything diet-related brought out a snotty jackass part of me. I didn't like or want to feel so petty inside, yet it happened often.)

After my initial, fairly short period of emaciation, I was never that skinny-skinny again. In fact, I gained a lot of pounds (a freaking lot—I couldn't fit into "average" sizes). Then I lost most of that weight and continued to bounce around between my extremes. My "maintenance" practices spanned from mild to severe methods, frequent to less frequent. Mostly, though, I looked "normal" in our society, and my constant dieting practices were normalized every day by advertisements, articles, and social conversations. I now realize that I would have qualified as having both clinical (meeting the actual diagnosis) and subclinical (problematic but not matching any diagnostic label) eating disorders throughout these decades.

Though I didn't believe myself to be in danger at any time, physical quirks happened that were likely a result of my "maintenance" practices. In addition to a regularly edgy mood and irregular sleep, I occasionally experienced a puffy face, dizziness, and feeling weirdly "off" inside my body. Usually, we don't feel or notice our insides or heartbeat; I definitely noticed mine at times. But I disregarded it all—except the puffy face that I frantically tried to de-puff because it looked strange.

Without telling my doctor about my "maintenance" practices, she didn't know to run the specific tests to check if I was safe inside. I'm randomly lucky that I didn't develop lasting or fatal health problems. My "off" feeling and my noticeable heartbeat could have been signs of electrolyte abnormalities, weakened heart, dehydration, or other serious issues. Thankfully, the body is forgiving and can often heal when the behaviors are corrected or stopped.

No matter what was going on inside me, I still appeared to be fine. In fact, people referred to me as a "high achiever." I consistently performed well in school, and from my first "real" job as a teen (a juicer in a juicery) to full careers, I excelled at work, too. However, my dieting, weight obsession, and body image issues ruled my days from my tweens into my thirties. Always present, their intensity and severity ebbed and flowed. Correspondingly, my contentment in life was limited and uneven.

I couldn't fully witness or participate in most things, because there was usually this humming or banging distraction. During my courting years, I romanced the bread on the table instead of my dinner dates. Celebrations all involved food and were usually more like scared-ebrations for me, like my friend's 30th birthday. Thankfully, she forgave me.

People tell me that I presented, for the most part, a free-spirited, full-of-life persona to the outside world during those years. But I was far from feeling free or full-of-life.

Why-Oh-Why Change?

You may be wondering; when food and body issues are that embedded—a way of existing—why and how does someone heal, change, or recover from them?

As a mental health professional and eating disorders specialist, I can wholeheartedly share that what each person wants to conquer and their journeys to do so are unique. For me, the birthday cake incident humiliated me, but it wasn't enough to make me challenge or change my "maintenance" practices. Instead, a bunch of other stuff lined up to help me realize that I wanted a different, more contented life—one with less focus on food, body, and weight.

Here's one of the most influential factors: anger. Though the feeling often takes a bad rap as a negative emotion, I think anger is awesomely informative. It's a waving red flag that broadcasts, "Hey, something is wrong! Since you're not acknowledging it, I'm going to get your attention!"

For years I had fastidiously kept photo albums. I finally noticed that when I looked back at decades of what others regarded as "cool" or "exciting" memories, I rarely recalled the event, my connections to the occasion, or the people in the photos. Who did I go to that formal with? Why did I meet that celebrity? How did I get talked into being on that parade float? Instead, I remembered my weight or dress size in each shot. This made me mad.

Simultaneously, I'd met someone special who would become the love of my life. I felt protective of being able to recall both present and future memories—and not by weight or size. Also, my parents were getting older, and I wanted clear recollections with them too.

Then one more significant thing happened to jolt me. Long after that cake episode, that same dear friend confronted me in a loving way. It went something like this: "I know you may get mad at me, and this could ruin our friendship, but I don't think what you're doing—your 'maintenance'—is normal. I don't think it's okay or healthy. I feel concerned about you." Of course I got outraged inside. But something about her bravery touched me. I must have been sufficiently open and the timing must have been right enough to hear it. Plus, I think the guilt I had from messing up her birthday helped me listen to her.

For years I'd been working with a really skilled generalist therapist, but I'd mostly kept the eating and weight stuff out of the room. I hadn't wanted her to know much about it or to meddle with it. After all, I'd accepted my "maintenance" practices as a forever part of my life.

Angry and fed up (no pun intended), at last, I said it: "I need accountability and help. Here's what I've been doing..." I wasn't scared when I told her. I felt calm, desperate, determined, and also relieved to stop hiding my secrets.

25

From Tripping Up a Path to Triumphing

At this point, I simply wanted my "maintenance" to occupy less time and space in my mind, be easier, and not take a toll on my body. I'd not been able to make those things happen. Change was needed, but what the heck was that going to be? I'd already tried every traditional diet and weight management method I knew.

Conquering my food, weight, and body image issues was messy and not at all linear. I'd experiment with something new, get frustrated with it, and give up, only to try again later. I'd commit to cutting down on or stopping the "maintenance" behaviors only to have to commit again the next day. I wish I could tell you which of my shifts was easiest or hardest; it was a bit of Whack-a-Mole. Once one thing got easy or I found my groove with it, the next "opportunity for growth" popped up. Sometimes I had to stay put for a while, take a break.

It took years to distill this information into a dozen shifts to offer to you. If even one supports you or starts you considering your own path towards a life you prefer, then that's meaningful for both you and me. And please don't think I did any of these conquering-methods with grace or ease, as they might imply due to their written brevity. For a long time, they seemed more like foundering-methods. I tripped and stumbled, awkwardly finding my way.

****

Beginning phase: your formula will evolve as yours, but here are four pieces I recall as being my helpful starters.

1. *I began to challenge the validity of my food beliefs and "maintenance" practices.* I asked myself, "Are fasting and purging really nutritionally sound?" I then found myself reviewing basic nutrition information and needing science. It was hard to figure out what offered real guidance since so many studies catered to supporting fad diets. I was already living *that* life and didn't want more of it. (If you crave science, there are some great sources in the Resources section of this book.)

2. *I needed to break my dieting and compensatory habits and replace them with a natural relationship with food.* I remember feeling dumb and vulnerable learning how to eat again. Observing people who had unstressed relationships with eating helped me. They'd unapologetically get a snack or stop activities for a meal. I did my best to copy them, even when it terrified me to eat what or as much as they did. Yet I found myself feeling more satisfied, energetic, and steady when I basically emulated their nutrition styles and schedules.

3. *I had to get honest with my medical doctor.* Complete with fear-tears, I asked her to run laboratory tests that pertained to extreme diets, strenuous exercise, and purging. Terrified after so many years of body mistreatment, I finally received the report. She had put a smiley face on it because nothing catastrophic was indicated.

Why didn't my body have gnarly damage? I don't know except that bodies are different. One person can die from complications related to a period of purging or severe food restriction whereas another may escape harm.

4. I had to find and execute healthier coping skills than bingeing, purging, dieting, and spending hours in the gym. I remember one seemingly ridiculous idea that helped a great deal. I hung index cards from long strings of tape in my cupboards and refrigerator. My hand would hit them as I reached for food, and my eyes couldn't miss the dangling cards. Each reminded me of ten things—e.g., go for a walk, swing the bat at the batting cages, paint my toenails, take a bath, write my thoughts in a journal, call a friend, sing a song, etc.—that I could do instead of eating when I wasn't actually hungry (for food, that is).

The first time I tried the "go for a walk" option, I made it to the front door of the apartment building, hastily tagged the green doorframe like a kid on a playground, and bolted back upstairs to binge. With enough attempts, I later made it all the way in a square-block. Eventually, I got myself to do five things first, each time. If the urge to binge was still there after completing the five, I binged. However, I usually didn't at that point.

Middle phase: these next five gained the most momentum during the in-between.

1. I had to learn to listen to my body and trust that it knows what's best. I was sure my first craving would be for something exciting. Nope. I heard "spinach" and thought, "How boring!" Yet it was accurate. Why? Because I had low iron at that time, so my craving was spot on. From that moment forward, I practiced listening to my body. Sometimes I could hear, sometimes I couldn't, but eventually, I became fantastic at it.

2. I needed to gain insight into life triggers that made me depend on my food, exercise, and dieting practices. I was fortunate to have that smart, caring therapist who helped me. FYI, none of this came as an instant realization. Although in time, I grew to understand previous triggers (the interactions and situations that used to catapult poor coping into action). Those realizations opened up different and better options.

3. I needed to find and use my voice. This meant doing what alarmed me: standing up for myself and saying "no." The Golden Rule is to treat others how I'd like to be treated. Since I wouldn't want to be hurt or disappointed by anyone, why would I *ever* want to hurt or disappoint someone? I believed this could bring on terrible consequences.

Okay, here's what I discovered. To be balanced, we need to know and say our limits. Boundaries do not equal bitchy; they translate into self-protection and safety. Interestingly, I'd been sure that the using-my-voice thing would make people not like me or see me as selfish. On the contrary, it brought people closer to me.

4. I had to learn to tolerate the gamut of emotions humans experience and cannot control. I liken feelings to the cans on the back of one of those "Just Married" 1950's cars. It drives along with the cans trailing, clanking behind. Slam on the brakes, and the cans smack into the back of the vehicle. Emotions I had avoided would inevitably smack into me in the same way. No matter how hard I tried, I couldn't make them vanish. They patiently waited, building up, ready to explode at whatever would be the tipping point. So I had to get the hang of labeling my feelings (not an easy task for many with eating issues), feeling them, accepting them, and allowing them to metabolize… or else, SMACK!

5. I needed accountability. I loved earning star-stickers from teachers when I was a kid. Goofy as this may sound, when I started my clumsy conquering of food, weight, and body issues, I kept a calendar; I put a star on each day that I didn't do any compensatory behaviors (purging, over-exercising, etc.). At some point, with enough rows of stars, I began to trust that I could get through the day without needing the physical star to mark the accomplishment. Bit by bit and day-by-day, the changes I made added up.

End phase: the in-between pieces eventually tumbled into these three.

1. I had to figure out who I was. I remember starting the process by making lists. What are my values? What do I value/not value in friends? A career? A partner? Knowing what's important to me helps to guide every day and decision. It gives a different and preferred meaning to looking in the mirror.

2. I had to accept myself, even what I didn't like. For example, I used to have quite a streak of jealousy. I despised that feeling. How could I possibly accept something so hideous within me? Well, I discovered that the ugly feeling of jealousy wasn't so ugly—it informed me. It meant that I wanted something someone else had. If I didn't DO anything bad with the feeling, like sabotaging someone or talking terribly about them, then it was just a feeling and not something inherently bad or shameful. So I let jealousy teach me when to work harder.

3. I had to thank my body instead of picking on it. Anytime I found myself focusing on a part of my body in a negative or hateful way, I'd shift to noticing the function and find appreciation for what it does. For example, my thighs let me sit and stand countless times a day. Get the picture?

****

With these dozen shifts, I was able to dump my "maintenance" and frenemies, meaning the unhelpful and unhealthful thoughts, diets, and behaviors that had kept me company for decades. This resulted in a pleasant surprise: my life grew, as did my memories and sense of purpose.

I think it's important to point out here that the process of making these changes could sound too self-focused to some people. On the contrary, getting free of my dieting and body struggles made me less self-focused and more available to support causes, do advocacy work, be present in relationships, and help others. Food, dieting, exercise, and calories no longer dominated conversations, which allowed for different, new, and dynamic interactions with people. Life got more interesting.

I stopped dreading social events because of the food and participated in living. At special celebrations, I'd enjoy a dessert—or two. Sometimes, I'd take a few bites and feel satisfied, done. I remember that different people kept saying, as if I had done something oddly remarkable, "How can you stop at just two bites?" I'd reply, "Because I'm done and happy," which I was. I felt such empathy for their responses. I also felt thankful for my non-stressed relationship with food.

I could look at a picture of myself and smile (or wince). I knew who was in it and why we took the shot. I had real memories of experiences instead of weight records.

With such a different, fuller, and more contented life, I gradually felt recovered, free from my dieting, weight, body issues, and even eating disorders. Without continuing to obsess about these topics, I had time and energy to spare. So I tried out different activities and interests.

While serving on an eating disorder recovery website, I realized that psychology ignited me and always had. I went back to school, became a licensed Marriage and Family Therapist, began presenting workshops and publishing in trade magazines, earned the designation of Certified Eating Disorders Specialist, and attained a second license.

I feel joy—an emotion that used to elude me—and gratitude for having created a movement called #ShakeIt for Self-Acceptance!® which sparks important conversations about body, soul, and self-acceptance through positivity and flash mob dance fun. It's my privilege to witness people accepting themselves, supporting each other, and abandoning judgment.

I'm not going to say that my life is "perfect" nowadays. Oh my gawd, it's not. Perfect isn't a destination anyway. But here's what I will say to you: life can be so much freaking better than it probably is right now for you (or you likely wouldn't be reading this).

Note from Alli:

I want to call attention to a few things from my story. Had I asked a professional about what I needed to do to fix my preoccupation with food and weight, I suspect I would've received this kind of advice: "Stop purging, find an appropriate eating plan, incorporate a good amount of exercise, and make sure that your weight falls within the BMI range." (I often hear about this sort of simplistic feedback given to people struggling.) In reality, I had to find the micro-steps I needed to eventually conquer my eating, weight, and body image issues. Through experiments, I started to find flickers of life-enhancing perspectives and practices. More happened, and so on. Nowadays, I feel thankful for having had those once-problems; they made me grow.

As my story shows, at the time, I sincerely felt I was doing the right things for my health and body with my "maintenance." Yet here's the truth I've since learned: long-term, or sometimes even short-term, manipulating what we eat, exercising too much, purging, and using other compensation methods, can damage one's body and quality of life. Unwitting consequences can include but are not limited to slowed metabolism (Ironic, huh? What the eff?), dull skin, and a bunch of other real, often serious medical issues related to hormones, the gastrointestinal tract, electrolytes, the heart, etc.

For many of us, if we knew those potentially safety-threatening risks came from something else (non-dieting, non-weight, or non-body-image-related), we'd probably openly seek the support of a medical professional, right? Yet when it comes to dieting, weight, and body image-related purposes, many of us do know about those risks. And yet we still spend each day with our safety possibly compromised. Why do you think that happens?

Although dieting is distinct from an eating disorder, dieting (for health or weight loss) is often a portal to an eating disorder. Science suggests that clinical eating disorders are caused by a combination of genetic and environmental factors. I had the magical mix to push the "on" button at different times. None of us know who has that button until it clicks on.

This story mentions harmful treatment that happened decades ago. Since the 1980s, thankfully, much has advanced in science to correct myths about eating disorders and health. Guidance about food and body image issues from a professional (who has been trained in those issues) can be extremely helpful nowadays.

Lastly, the Storytellers and I are sharing our personal life-experiences with you, and for some (like me), dieting should have come with a warning label. I can't predict how your choices relating to food, weight, and body image will affect you. Yet I can share this: the absolute thinking (all good/all bad) that's common in the realms of eating and health often isn't helpful and may be downright problematic, creating obstacles in the way of your conquering. An open mind and curiosity about what might truly support you, what can help you to overcome your struggles, will be most beneficial.

DISCOVERIES

THE STORIES IN THIS SECTION, "Discoveries," answer, "How _____ is different now that I don't struggle with my food, weight, and body image issues." I couldn't resist filling in the blank: "How I use my personality traits is different now that I don't struggle."

Personality traits (e.g., perfectionistic, empathetic, laid-back, etc.) are basically the ingredients that make up any human's distinct way of being. No two people can be exactly alike since no combination of these will be exactly the same.

People often tell me they notice my persistence and attention to detail. Listing those characteristics on a job resume, both seem positive. Yet during my eating issues, these seemingly favorable attributes damaged my wellbeing. The persistence helped me to commit to undereating for extended periods, which resulted in normal human responses of crankiness and rigidity. The attention to detail helped me to track calories in an overly specific, burdensome way (e.g., estimating for toothpaste calories that I might have swallowed).

As an eating disorders specialist, I've asked clients/patients (I prefer the term "people"), "What are two personality traits it takes to be good at having an eating disorder?" I pose the same question to you but ask you to replace "eating disorder" with whatever your issue is.

- "What are two personality traits it takes to be good at having [your issue]?"

- Think about it.

- Got your two? Please hold onto them for later.

People frequently answer my question with seemingly negative characteristics such as "manipulative" and "controlling." That's okay. Our personality traits are like the superpowers that heroes or villains have—how one *uses* the superpower determines whether it's beneficial or destructive.

If eating or body image issues are in charge, "manipulative" can mean that you get loved ones to accept what you say, agree to rules they don't actually support, and fulfill requests they don't want to fulfill (e.g., relating to food shopping, scheduling, exercising, and so on.). However, let's look at the helpful side of manipulative. Doesn't it also mean *persuasive*—someone who gets others to agree to or back something? Isn't this a strong and desirable trait in many situations like advocacy work, politics, and sales? How we use manipulative/persuasive behavior makes it positive or negative.

When influenced by eating or body issues, being "controlling" may mean that you successfully organize others around your food and exercise rituals. Digging deeper, taking control can be a tremendous aid in life. It can mean that you ably create organization for yourself and others, which is most helpful when a leader is needed.

Remember those two traits you picked? Please go back to them and explore their harmful and helpful sides.

While immersed in my food, weight, and body-related issues, I used my superpowers in self-destructive ways. Once I did the work to free up that tenacity and meticulousness, each could be applied for my benefit or the benefit of others. Nowadays, I pour both into things that feel important in life—like this book.

Here, I must give credit to Carolyn Costin,[4] my first clinical director. She introduced me to the idea of personality features manifesting as assets or liabilities, and I witnessed that the concept could make a powerful difference in how we see ourselves.

Try getting to know more of your personality traits, the helpful and harmful sides of each. Even a slight shift in how you view or use a superpower can help you to

---

[4] Costin, *About Carolyn*, (2018).

overcome your issues and to claim more of your brimming, meaningful life.

Never Going to be Perfect

Anonymous

THE BABY WANTED "junk food." Every day.

I ballooned up during my pregnancy because I didn't crave celery. I craved cookies and ice cream, the same things that I denied myself while I danced professionally. After the birth, I planned to resume my normal eating and go back to my dancing as usual.

I'm a petite, curvy, half Japanese woman who spent the first part of my life performing next to six feet tall, ultra-thin dancers with legs up to my shoulders. Because the professional world of dance placed so much focus on a dancer's looks, shape, and weight, I had to work extra hard to get jobs amid those girls. Fortunately, I kept getting hired because I loved to dance, I'm good at it, and I worked my ass off.

However, the costumes were usually geared towards slim, long-legged women; they didn't look good on me. In this one vertically striped unitard, the other girls showed

41

three stripes across the thigh. Me? Five. When I split the butt of a different costume, I got a write-up; the dance captain told me to lose weight. I felt shocked and concerned that I might get fired because the old satin bottoms had worn thin in the rear and ripped. I had already *lost* weight since the beginning of that show. It was so unfair!

Daily, I desired that unachievable, unattainable, tall and thin body that, at the time, permeated the dance industry. Even when I got skinny, I still had hips because my bones are shaped that way. My boobs sunk in. I accepted, "This is just how I am."

I disliked my genetic imprint. I disliked me.

An extra hard work ethic helped me to repeatedly manage the body loathing that dominated the first half of life, as well as the emotional eating that heavily influenced the second part, which you'll now see.

Suddenly and without warning, my world flipped on its axis. I gave birth to this infant whose unexpected prognosis devastated me. My boy was likely not going to live for even a year and had received a provisional diagnosis of cerebral palsy. My existence played like a country song: in a short period of time, my husband left, my mom passed away from cancer, and my cat got eaten by a coyote.

Extraordinarily alone as I was, my seizing baby needed me 24/7. I loved him so much, and I didn't want him to die. I tried to manage his care, see all the recommended specialists, handle what became an expensive and long divorce, deal with the heartbreak of losing my mom and cat, and just get through each day.

Food wound up as my only comfort because I didn't have anybody to hug me. I didn't have anybody or anything that felt solid. I couldn't put a nipple on a vodka bottle, sit in the back of my closet, and hide from everyone. Smoking pot would have left me too impaired. So whenever I felt overwhelmed and very alone—both happened often—I turned to food for solace and as my friend.

Cookies were heaven. I remember I had been living at the hospital while my son had pneumonia. After his fifth consecutive admission, I questioned if he was going to pull through. After I finally got to bring him home, I went to the store. As a relief and a reward, I bought two bags of cookies and mindlessly ate.

To bring you now to the present, it has been 18 years since his birth. My son is debilitated, but he is alive. My stressors have been constant, and most of these years, I have been an "emotional eater."

Not too long ago, I realized that stress and emotional eating had taken a toll on my health; I received some medical diagnoses. At nearly 60, this news shocked me into choosing health over emotional eating, body image, and stuff like that. Of course, I still sometimes feel overwhelmed and devastated, like when my son is sick and might die, or he's in pain that I can't fix, but I handle it differently now.

To begin to change the emotional eating, I first had to stabilize my life. This meant getting used to it and accepting whatever it was. Then, I had to make some time for me. Enlisting nursing to aid with my son's 24/7 care helped, but even that took around eight years before I could begin to power down.

I gradually found my freedom from both my emotional eating and that preexisting body loathing through looking inside, learning, and changing. Here are the main components that I found to be my fixes. I hope that some might support you, too.

****

Ask for help.

I had to be able to ask for help, which is hard for me, an independent woman. What was the alternative? Sitting there in the depths of grief. Eating. Staying stuck in that awful, awful place.

I sucked at relationships. So I never got support from a romantic partner, but I got it in spades when it came to friends. There were days I'd pick up the phone. My friend would say, "Hello." Trying not to cry, I couldn't talk. Silence. He knew it was me from caller ID, and he'd say, "Doll, what do you need?" Silence. "Do you need to come over?" I'd croak, "Yes." He'd say, "Tell me when." Me: "Tomorrow afternoon." He'd say, "Okay." And that was it. He'd hang up.

Sometimes I just needed somebody to care. I was so overwhelmed and not handling it. They, the people I reached out to, gave me love. Asking for their support got me through some of the hardest times.

Find a mentor.

I found a therapist who specialized in services for family members with disabilities. She helped me traverse the systems that could assist with my son's disability. She understood how to navigate the bureaucratic shit that is part of life, and she became my advocate. Her support helped put Humpty Dumpty back together again.

Open up.

I opened myself to everything I could find that might help—alternative medicine, healers, anything.

Eat mindfully.

I wasn't feeling great. My moods and energy were crap. Wanting to feel better and improve my health pushed me into being more mindful about eating, taking pleasure in food, and honoring both cravings and what I'm needing for nourishment.

Include contentment in your life.

To me, contentment is that feeling of being centered in my life. Through mindful eating and acquiring the practices of meditation and gratitude, I brought more contentment into my life.

Meditate.

I had no idea if it would help, but I kept doing free meditations I found online. This really alleviated my stress and increased my awareness as far as gratitude was concerned.

I still don't know *why* the meditations helped so much. I just know that after about a week of practicing them, I was driving around and I noticed I felt happy, fulfilled, and grateful. I wondered, "What the hell? Where did this come from?" I felt better.

Identify what you're grateful for.

While grasping for things to hold onto, something Oprah said on her talk show struck me. She spoke about writing daily in a gratitude journal. I started one. I wrote in that sucker every day the year my son was born. It did not make everything better, but it helped. Forced to find a few things to be thankful for, I started building this habit of trying to find gratitude in any given instant.

After all these years, I still make sure I have a moment each day where I give thanks, and it can be for whatever. When I'm driving to dance class, I may thank God (for me it's God, but for you, it might be different) for this beautiful day and that my body is healthy enough to take a dance class.

My whole perspective has changed. I went to another country four years ago. The public toilet was a porcelain hole and a bucket of water with a scoop to flush. When I gave my porter a tip, he said, "I'm going to use this money to buy electricity." Electricity? I thought, "Oh my God. I have *so much*."

I realized that some of my eating, stress, and body-loathing stuff had been about feeling a "lack," believing that I don't have abundance in my life. But I do. I have more than I need.

Here's the shocking conclusion I've reached. Mitigating my stress is not about eating. Mitigating my stress is about meditating, exercising, getting outside, spending time with friends, and cuddling my cat. It can be about advocating for my family and myself when it's needed, even if that means battling hospitals and medical bureaucratic monsters. For me, it's about finding and maintaining a space of gratitude.

****

Steel is forged in fire. Walking through the fire of my life, I grew stronger and learned to look at my world in a way I may have otherwise missed. The feel of my son's velvety cheek, the sun on my face, and a book in my lap—these are perfect moments. When I am truly living in these instants and not in the "I need to be at the grocery store, then at the—" I am more than okay.

Shit's never going to be perfect. But we, you and me, can notice and appreciate a moment of perfection—like laughing your butt off with a friend; it's *in that moment*. And those moments add up to a level of contentment.

The one thing that keeps me away from both emotional eating and body loathing is gratitude. You cannot treat yourself cruelly while in the midst of gratitude.

Note from Alli:

When you think of remedies for body hate and emotional eating, what comes to your mind? Many of us probably go to what seems logical regarding dissatisfaction with the body—change the body to dislike it less. Advice to correct emotional eating? That often includes controlling the food intake, removing tempting items from the house, and increasing discipline. Unfortunately, those methods can be unreliable. Instead, our Storyteller learned to use different, personally effective, maintainable practices. Her shifts in attitude and actions helped her to heal from body hate and emotional eating while also enriching her life.

I want to mention "junk food" here because exploring our preconceived notions can be part of our conquering expedition. With that said, I ask you: what if having "junk food" as we desired it instead of forbidding it might prevent a later episode of emotionally eating, overeating, or bingeing it? This might not be for everyone, but for some, the food then loses its power over us. That sounds useful, not junky at all.

Among the components described in this narrative, our Storyteller points out the practice of meditation as a distinct turning point for her. There are different ways to meditate, and the benefits of it have been well-documented (may reduce stress, alleviate anxiety, increase ability to relax, and so on). If you feel curious about meditation, an accessible overview of research can be found in the online article, "Meditation: In Depth," by the National Center for Complementary and Integrative Health.[5]

If you've already tried meditation and it didn't work for you, that's okay! But before you cross it off the list completely, I encourage you to ask yourself: "Did I practice a form that I could connect with?" and "Did I try it for long enough?" The same questions apply to gratitude practices and any other conquering approach you may test. Here's why.

If something resonates—or could resonate—with you, then you're more likely to do it than if it didn't. You might even want to eventually adopt it as a part of your lifestyle. About duration, while researching an article I was writing, I read a lot about habits and the brain. I discovered that contrary to popular belief, there seems to be no "'X' number of days" that assures the formation of a habit. It can require more time and attempts than anticipated. With an open mind and inquisitiveness, you'll likely notice if and when changes happen for you.

When emotional eating has become a primary coping skill, it can feel impossible to stop. Instead, try adding methods to help you cope, like those in this story. Use a skill or two—maybe a few—**before** going to your emotional

---

[5] National Center for Complementary and Integrative Health, *Meditation: In Depth*, (2016).

eating. The more skills you can enlist, the less you may need to rely on emotional eating as a mainstay.

The Journey

Shannon Hershkowitz

BEATEN DOWN AND in tears, filled with feelings of worthlessness—I spent more than 25 years this way. I thought everyone would be better off without me. Memories of the abuse still haunt me.

My childhood was filled with love, laughter, and adventure. In the middle of the Chickahominy River, my sister and I would flip our small sailboat to hide under it together. Whether we were dodging imaginary pirates or scoping for sharks, you could hear our hushed giggles from the shore. Life was delightful then.

As a teenager, my home, my safe place broke. When I stood close to my father, I began to notice an occasional smell—alcohol. He also started to disappear. My mother, who worked full-time, seemed to grow overwhelmed, stressed, and full of rage at times. They fought, loud screaming. Desperate to be independent, find peace, and feel free, I left home at 17.

Fearless, I blew like the wind in my red Jeep Wrangler—the breeze whipping through my hair, my destination: *anywhere.* I had no agenda and no one to answer to. I slept in my car and showered in truck stops. I ate from fruit stands on the side of backcountry roads. I can still taste those sweet, juicy peaches.

After about four years of this freedom, a simple life of hanging out with myself, exploring the world, and experiencing so many beautiful souls, moments, and settings… *I pull into a small town in Arizona: population of about 3,000 people, one stop light, and horses have the right of way. I arrive confident, strong, and fierce. Here, I see him— the prince that I dreamt about growing up. I remember little me, in my tree fort, imagining him—THIS man—on his white horse, riding up to greet me. He whispers my name as I walk by him at a local bank. (It's a small town, and everyone knows everyone.) He takes my breath away. My heart renders a soft patter of approval. He is kind. Life is going to be great. I know it. I stay put, for him, in this little town in Arizona.*

After dating for two years, we married in the front yard of a ranch, standing in the morning dew. A gentle touch and a soft kiss sealed our commitment to each other—so much love between my fairytale prince and me.

Learning how to work as husband and wife challenged both our patience with each other and our communication skills. Nonetheless, I knew that together, we could do anything. Being with him calmed my spirit; I no longer wanted the fierce independence. I preferred togetherness and love—a home.

Then just about nine months after our wedding and with the most beautiful baby boy in my arms, my world changed. Grateful to expand that home with family, I put all my time, energy, and love into our son and a few years later, our daughter. I gave to my husband where I could, and working full-time demanded my attention, too. I lost myself. (Hear what I didn't say? I didn't say that I "let myself go.")

Everything I had known vanished, especially my independence and freedom. For years, I couldn't even take a shower alone without a child with me! Exhausted, with nothing left to give, my hair went up and makeup came off. I owned yoga pants and sweatpants in every color. Oversized clothing replaced my fitted, cute wardrobe. Stains, holes, and dryer-wrinkles were fine, as long as I covered my body. Sleepless nights, carpools, homework, school plays, and fast food became normal. "Cereal for dinner, anyone?"

I wanted to run away at times, drive as fast as I could, back to when life was simple. Back to those long, winding dirt roads.

As my body changed, I felt sure I saw the disappointment in my prince's eyes. To get back the svelte woman he married on that spring day, I tried every diet, detox, and exercise regimen: Jenny Craig, Cabbage Soup Diet, Metabolife, Atkins Diet, HCG Diet, The Master Cleanse, and more. I took laxatives and diuretics. Everything would be perfect if I were just thin. I'd be happy and have energy. I'd be a better mom and wouldn't yell at my kids so much. My husband would desire me again.

Here's where I got into a relationship with the abuser: me. I was my own victim. Days of eating light or nothing at all spiraled into binges that would lead me to the toilet. "Please God, let me throw up, I want to have bulimia." I'd pray this as my sweet babies knocked on the door, "Mama, are you okay?" I'd holler, "Yes, I'll be out in a minute!" I felt angry that I did not have the willpower to be successful at any eating disorder—I couldn't *not* eat for long, and I couldn't get myself to easily vomit. Repeatedly, I'd berate myself, "I am such a failure."

Standing at the mirror with tears streaming down my face, I'd look at myself with sheer disgust. "What in the hell happened?!" I'd cry for the former woman who turned heads and was admired for her zest for life. *How* could my body produce two miracles *and* leave me looking like *this*? And if I hated how I looked, how then could he, my prince, love me?

For years, I abused myself with these kinds of words. I missed so many family meals, only to succumb later to a secret trip to any fast food drive-through, after which, the evidence disappeared. And the baked goods that my little angel made with so much love and wanted her mama to taste? I'd spit them out when she turned away. (This still hurts to remember.)

Self-hate.

To cope with these intense feelings about me/my body, I traveled to a faraway and dark place called *isolation*. I felt safe there and free of judgment. When anyone called to do something social, I said either, "Thank you, but I have to work," or "I'll certainly try," when I knew damn well that I wouldn't. I pushed away my kids and husband, too. "Mom, are you okay?" "Honey, do you want to talk?" No and no.

On the other hand, I also wore the most beautiful mask to cover my pain and keep the isolation a secret to outsiders: one of service. I was THE BEST at taking care of others—codependency at its finest! "What can I do for you today?" "How can I help?" "Sorry family, I can't go to dinner because I have to help out at...." I had to stay in control, but I caught myself asking, "Am I really in control?"

Life continued to move forward. Despite abusing myself and teeter-tottering from service to isolation, I was a good mom. At least, I tried hard to be. I kept my kids active in the community. They played instruments, chased balls, and shouted cheers while pumping up the crowd. They were happy, kind, and animal lovers. "Mom, I just want to bring him home so you can hold him" suckered us into more than one pet. Teachers, store clerks, and just about any adult told me how respectful they were. Yep, we did good.

Still trying to find the solution to master my body image hate, I continued with my fad diets. Then, out of nowhere, *it* happened...

55

"Mom, I hate my body!"

I freeze. It takes me a minute as I frantically try to find my breath. WHAT?! HOW? You're young and your body is flawless! What in the hell?! Damn you society! But wait... I feel a touch on my shoulder as I ask myself, "Did I teach her this? Did I fail at protecting my children from this self-hate-hell?"

I want to jump up and down, scream, and wave flags. DETOUR! You may not follow me down this road!

Now, I'm panicking. I must protect her, but how? How can I teach her about body acceptance when I feel like I'm dying inside from non-body acceptance? I tell her what to do. (I'm a mom, and I'm great at telling my children what they should do.) I authoritatively command: "Do not talk bad about your body! Say something nice."

She says, "Well, YOU do it." My spit freezes. Rage fills me.

I do not want to do it, but to save my children, I would fight a hundred Goliaths. Feeling pressured, I push out something ridiculous like "My shoes are cute." Exasperated, I then blurt, "Go to your room."

I needed to change my ways.

****

I battled to break my habit of commenting negatively on my body around my kids and then around me, too.

I did this first by becoming aware of when I did it. I'd catch myself mid-sentence and stop. Or I'd say the negative thing, and then I'd make myself say two positives—even when I was alone. That first attempt with my daughter had indicated I needed to improve at role modeling and naming those good things.

In our house, this evolved into the practice of "affirm yourself." If anything self-deprecating slipped out of our mouths, we had to say two positive things.

There were good and bad days, but I didn't give up. The comments grew to how pleasing my smile is and how much I love my eyes. I still remember the day when my daughter heard me say, unsolicited, "Wow, I feel pretty today." With a teeth-showing smile, she jumped off the bed and wrapped me up in a warm hug. "You look incredible, Mama." What an amazing feeling!

Other changes that helped to break my body image hate were these (not in order of importance since they all were vital).

I began to sit down at meal times with my family; we engaged in conversations and eventually laughter.

Of course at first, I was tense and not natural at this. Thankfully, my family is very talkative, and I'd try to join in the topic of the day to take my mind off eating. I realized I'd lost *how* to eat. There were many times that all I could do was to "match" someone: when my child took a bite, so did I. (I could never match my husband. I'd end up with indigestion. He inhales his food!) Family dinners helped me to form a different relationship with meals; they eventually became about nourishment and connection instead of rules and isolation.

I talked with my husband, scary as that was.

I learned that the disappointment I thought I saw in his eyes was my own judgment, not his. I had blamed my body's changes for the decrease in our intimacy. The real culprit? *Exhaustion.* We can laugh now about the times he'd get a very clear (sometimes non-verbal) communication: "You want me to do what? I don't think so!"

I had to figure out what self-care could look like for me.

A hot bath, intentionally scheduling "me" time, avoiding toxic people, good music, tidying up, blogging, any form of art... and especially time outside. This could be a long hike, feeling the sun kiss my shoulders and breathing in the mountains' fresh air, or just a trip to the front yard, a couple of deep breaths, feeling the grass, and listening to a bird's sweet song. Each reset and refueled me.

My daughter started to join me outside, and I noticed changes in her, too. "Mom, I feel great today." We both started to realize that *feeling great* came from connection with nature, each other, and movement—not the mirror.

Body acceptance naturally seemed to sneak in when these other aspects of life were full and present.

****

Nowadays, I feel at peace in my body and I always feel strong. Of course, sometimes I will look at myself, laugh, and tell that woman in the mirror, "Dang, you look like hell." When I have those moments, I do affirmations or self-care. My favorite, though, is to head straight to the trails. Nature is my safe place where I can feel that familiar sense of freedom and independence again. The sounds of the outdoors and the rhythm of my feet soothe me. Whether I fasten a heavy pack on my back or simply hold a water bottle, I appreciate the strength and power of this body that carries me miles into Mother Nature. The sound of my breath and my fast heartbeat remind me that I'M ALIVE! I AM FREE from the hell of body hate and self-abuse that comes with it.

I can't say that I *love* the look of all my body. I'm not sure if that would even be realistic with how our society is set up. But what I can say is this: I respect my body. I love what it does for me and the adventures it takes me on. I only have one, and I have much gratitude towards it for never giving up on me. It takes care of me, and for the rest of my life, I will do the same.

I used to diet and change my body to find myself. Instead, I got more lost than I had ever been. Are you lost? Are you abusing yourself, too? If you're breathing, it's not too late to work towards body acceptance. In a world where you can be anything you want, be your own friend.

Note from Alli:

Our Storyteller, Shannon, tried to get back to her before-she-became-a-mother body—so much so, she said that she abused herself both emotionally and physically. Instead of continuing down that path, she discovered humane, sustainable behaviors and views that helped her to overcome her body hate and yo-yo dieting (also known as weight cycling). These changes allowed her to leave her abusive relationship with herself.

Contrary to how it can feel in the moment, communal meals can be helpful and healing for people who struggle with disordered eating. If you have difficulty consuming food with (or in front of) other people, I invite you to create a list of conversation starters and questions. Hint: make sure you're INTERESTED in the topics because an ability to balance your attention on people *and* have an ease with eating can take time and practice.

In this story, Shannon attempted to use vomiting, laxatives, and diuretics as weight management tools. Caution! These methods can lead to internal imbalances that may not be felt and cannot be seen. These imbalances can then lead to—and have led to—cardiac arrest and death.

About the references made to the soothing and reparative power of nature, science supports this notion. If you want to check out some research, the following online articles can get you started: "Stanford Researchers Find

Mental Health Prescription: Nature," by Rob Jordan;[6] and "Sour Mood Getting You Down? Get Back to Nature," posted in Harvard Men's Health Watch.[7] If you haven't tried hanging out with Mother Nature—hiking, walking, sitting still and experiencing the outdoors with your senses—see if it's a tool you might add to your conquering toolbox.

---

[6] Jordan, *Stanford Researchers Find Mental Health Prescription: Nature*, (2015).

[7] Harvard Health Publishing, *Sour Mood Getting You Down? Get Back to Nature*, (2018).

My Inner World Was a Thunderstorm

Jaynie M. Goldberg

I DID NOT have an "off" button until my late 20's. My inner world was a thunderstorm. *In a fit of rage, I gathered years of keepsake letters and bracelets from my best friend, tossed it all in a big garbage bag, and left it on her front porch.*

You see, I valued my friends, but I could not tolerate things that I interpreted as betrayals. If a friend genuinely had other plans and could not hang out with me, I took this personally. I would feel abandoned and react in anger instead of understanding.

Childhood was all about managing my emotions. *Desperate to feel accepted, I once did homework for a classmate and gave him the better of two essays.*

I did not know what "good enough" meant. *When a bunch of us got A's, my teacher would point out and praise one person's work. Inside, I would explode if it wasn't me. I needed to do the best in the class, or I was a failure.*

During puberty, everything was awkward. I felt different from others. Less than. I focused on looks as the fix. *I wanted to get contacts to make my brown eyes green because the people with those characteristics didn't seem insecure. I researched surgery on hair follicles to find out if I could make my black curly hair straight. The people with straight hair and blue or green eyes got complimented. If I had those things, maybe I would get compliments, too.*

My smarts intermittently and temporarily calmed my unrest during those angst-filled young years. At age 11 and with my parents' blessing, I started and ran a small, homemade greeting card business. This anchored me, knowing I was both creative and intelligent. I didn't totally suck.

Then in 8th grade, validation from boys became paramount and remained so until young adulthood. *While sitting on the playground in gym class, a friend shared a secret: "This is what guys want. People who are open to doing sexual acts, blowjobs, and stuff. That would make him want you." A light bulb went on in my head. I thought, "If boys would want me to do that, then they would have to want me. For that to happen, I would need to have a great body and to be pretty." I panicked. I realized that this smart, chunky geek was not going to be wanted, accepted. But, I could work on my body.*

By 14 years old, something had taken over. It started with consuming fewer calories. I knew that what I ate directly impacted the size of my body. Therefore, if I could eat less, my body would be smaller. I moved to trying to induce vomiting. For hours, I would hang over the toilet, attempting and failing.

Exercise grew to eight or more hours a day. In my room, I had two fitness machines. If it were dark or icy outside, I would glide on the elliptical and then ride the stationary bike—glide then ride, again and again. If it were light outside and clear weather, I would repeatedly run my routes in the neighborhood or rollerblade in circles in the backyard. I refused to go out with friends because I had to work out.

Nobody seemed to think any of this was a problem. At least, no one said so.

In college, I even took ipecac, the emetic (inducing-vomit) drug reported to have factored into Karen Carpenter's death. *We had to make first aid kits for a class, and that excuse to buy ipecac thrilled me. I feared using it—that it could harm or kill me, but I felt desperate.*

Ipecac was the worst experience for me—horrific stomach cramps, nausea, and vomiting. I used it twice.

All the while, I looked like a typical student to onlookers. During university, I kept up my grades, was active in a sorority, and partied a lot. Many of us compared notes on how we balanced alcohol calories by eliminating food. My sorority sisters ate dry bread before a heavy drinking night to help absorb the alcohol. I ate lettuce.

I still don't know *why* I needed constant reassurance that someone was attracted to me. I just could not hold onto it on my own. *I got pulled out of boys' rooms a lot by my older sorority sisters. People thought I was a slut. I was trying to be accepted and to connect, and that was how I chose to do it. I wanted to be close, and the boys expected more. There were times when I was in over my head; I didn't even remember what happened.*

I went out with so many guys—mostly for attention and partly because I felt obligated. Even if I didn't like them and wasn't attracted to them, I did not want to hurt their feelings. I knew how terrible that felt.

Besides the room extrications, no one, including me, seemed to see anything wrong. I continued keeping up my grades and showed up smiling at social activities. Some noticed and commented on my weight repeatedly fluctuating, but who didn't yo-yo? I don't think I had any friends during high school, college, or young adulthood who didn't participate in dieting or expressing dissatisfaction with their own bodies. As a matter of fact, they praised how much I exercised and how I would fit it around my class schedule.

The difference between my admiring friends or sorority sisters and me is that I had an eating disorder: bulimia nervosa. (I did not realize that until much later in my life.) I still don't know the *exact* cause of it, but cause is hard to pin down even in scientific research. It was probably a combination of temperament, genetics, teen hormones, and other internal and external stuff. I would still like to know for my own edification and closure, but in the end, a cure trumps the cause.

In retrospect, I partly understand why I maintained the behaviors for so many years (besides that I had an illness that makes it extremely difficult to stop them). Much more than being about boys and a preoccupation with my body, I believe my behaviors helped manage (although poorly) my out-of-control emotions. They kept me distanced from people who could deeply hurt me. They gave me a focus to channel my energy, confusion, anger, and vulnerabilities. My exercising gave me something to do so I wouldn't have to sit with my thoughts or emotions. When I felt about a five or six out of ten for my out-of-control feelings, I exercised, and it seemed to somewhat distract and calm me.

I have since learned that restricting, purging, and exercising affect the brain's chemistry, which means they impact mood, thinking, and feelings. I'm sure that my younger self was self-medicating through my behaviors—helping me avoid (or at least disrupt) natural emotions that I was not yet equipped to handle. The true irony I've discovered: my dieting, starving, bingeing, and excessive exercising likely *caused* more of those negative emotions and experiences, the same ones I was trying to avoid feeling. (Think about when you experience being angry or irritable because of hunger.)

My less than profound "aha" moment happened in the midst of compulsive running. I thought, "This sucks. How can things be different?" From there, it was slow, and if I had not avoided professional help, I think it would have been a much quicker repair.

Here are some actions I took that helped me. If you are feeling trapped in a diet, exercise, or a binge cycle of any severity, they might help you, too.

****

I started to consciously listen to the way I talked to and about myself.

I spoke back, challenged, and changed the narrative. If I heard the internal, "I'm not good enough," I would look for evidence to counter the thought. If I heard, "I cannot eat this," I would use logic to remind myself, for example, "I'll be hungry if I don't, and I should take care of my body."

I looked for and found realizations that mattered to me.

I noticed my attachment to weight/body image was my own construct. The way people responded to me depended on how I presented myself, not on my weight. For example, when I acted bitchy (which happened often, due to hunger or the pressure of my beliefs and behaviors), it was the bitchiness, rather than my weight, that brought on upsetting interactions.

I tapered down the over-exercising to more normal exercising.

I started giving myself permission: "I'm going to exercise a half-hour only, and that's going to be enough. An urge does not give me permission to add more activity." I became okay with doing *enough*.

I stopped restricting my food.

This helped me stop bingeing.

I quit partying.

This change was a result of circumstances more than any insight, but it was a good one nonetheless. I graduated and it was no longer easy to party. My job became more important.

I decided I was good enough.

Even if I had to "fake it 'till you make it" for a while, it became real.

I got in touch with my values.

I realized that my behaviors had gotten in the way of what was *truly* important to me. Acceptance and connection happened through eating a meal with my future husband, being with him, talking, or just watching a movie together.

****

I am still a perfectionist, can have strong emotional reactions, like to feel in control, and prefer (but don't need) to be accepted. I now value looking, being, and feeling different from others. I love my smarty-pants, inner geek. All these parts help make me "me."

I am happily married, healthy, and fully appreciate my body. I'm in a powerful position in my career, in love with my kids, and feel overall contented with life.

I have self-esteem issues sometimes, but who doesn't?

My inner thunderstorm rarely happens now, and it's more like a quick sprinkle or shower when it does. No matter what the internal weather, I know that it's all going to pass. My father's tragic, sudden, and unexpected death as a result of an illness could have broken me at 34. Instead, I was (and sometimes still am) an appropriately grief-stricken, sad mess.

We are all human, and sometimes we have big emotions. It's okay to feel.

Note from Alli:

In this story, Jaynie shares that she began losing weight to become attractive to boys. Many of us have probably done something similar in wanting to attract a partner. As we know, recommendations for weight loss usually include restricting food intake and exercising more (the familiar "calories in, calories out" equation). Jaynie was already doing a lot of both. And though her compulsive dieting and exercise had morphed into a disorder, along with those around her, she simply continued to live in a world of diet culture (societal prizing of thinness). Eventually, through dieting less, exercising less, altering behaviors, and gaining awareness, Jaynie found her personal route to triumph over her food and body image issues. Her problems helped her find outlooks and actions that enhanced her life.

Often, when a person has a strong desire for weight loss, they won't assess danger or threat to themselves accurately. For example, Jaynie believed that trying ipecac could hurt her or cause her death; she tried it anyway. Twice. An "It won't happen to me" or "It's not THAT bad" kind of minimization or disconnection can be present. Consequently, the person's rational brain, reasoning, and risk assessment may be less reliable than usual.

If you're someone dead set on losing weight, could that be true for you? (And if you love someone who might have an eating disorder, be cautious about assuming "They'd never do that" or "They know better"—especially if the topic is anything related to food, body, or weight. Chances are they would and they don't.) Jaynie shared that she "avoided professional help." Especially since the behaviors referenced in this piece can be dangerous, professional support would be advised.

This story is the first after mine to mention an eating disorder. Knowing the characteristics of diagnoses can help you to notice if dieting or health practices may have developed into a disorder. For example, Jaynie identified with having bulimia nervosa. Yet she couldn't make herself throw up except twice from the ipecac syrup. Her primary behaviors were restricting and exercising, which can constitute a less recognized form of bulimia nervosa. In our diet-focused culture, disordered behaviors can be difficult to spot.

70

Jaynie indicated that values helped her solve her problems. Here's an exercise you might find beneficial.

- What are some of your core values? If you're not sure, ask yourself, "What's important to me in myself, in others, and in life? For example, honesty, kindness, being popular, etc. Get the picture?

- Make a list of your values. Go ahead and free-flow it, writing down whatever pops into your mind.

- Thoughtfully review the words you chose, what they mean to you, and what priority each holds.

- Whittle the list down to the ten you value most. Try removing any appearance-related core values.

- Then arrange them in order of importance to you. What are your top three to five?

- When you have choices to make or you're figuring out if a person/environment is a good fit in your life, consult your list.

Knowing your values helps you to make empowering decisions, including those related to conquering food, weight, and body image issues.

Take the Body I'm Giving You

Anonymous

AFTER A 35-PLUS-YEAR career as a singer, touring with famous headliners, I finally got called in and called out about my body. My boss said pointed, personal, and ugly things about me. It was the most humiliating, horrible experience of my career.

I started like many young, aspiring creative-arts people—taking any job where I could be me and use my skills. In my 20s, I found real people modeling, which was a gas! It's a category of modeling where the models are supposed to look like an average Joe or an ordinary Jane. I was muscular, not tall, and didn't look like Naomi Campbell; I looked like me. I ended up representing corporations all over the United States as the girl next door with an Afro.

To make ends meet, I also taught voice to kids, sang in a band, and did random gigs for an event company. My musical group had just settled into a permanent job when a friend encouraged me to audition for a tour. A Grammy-award winning artist I loved was seeking backup vocalists. I figured, "Why not?"

I drove many hours to reach that audition, and of hundreds, they picked two of us. This happened decades ago, and work as a vocalist has stayed steady since then. Yes, people have sometimes treated me unfairly or poorly (you know, the bullshit), but I'm a resilient person. It's in my DNA and has been fantastic armor. For instance, I remember working with this one choreographer who had a problem with me. There were around 12 of us, and he singled me out *every* time we practiced the number. In the middle of the song, only I would get "notes" (feedback and corrections about the work). I'd smile and say, "Got it," when I wanted to say instead, "Jesus Christ. Just let us do it once without stopping to correct me!"

Since receiving "notes" is simply part of the job, I always need to be professional about them. (I can explode later over a beer with my best friend.) I've been trained not to personalize these corrections and criticisms, and when I've made the mistake of personalizing them, I've learned I can't get past them. So I've made it a point to untether my ego and always ask myself two questions: (1) "Are they right about that?" and (2) "Is there something that I can learn from this?"

In the case of the choreographer, after I excavated answers to my questions, I was able to start reassuring myself: "This is not about me, this is about him," which got me through the rest of that job with my sanity intact.

I've seen people get hired and fired a lot. On more than one gig or tour, I've come back from lunch and been surprised, "Oh man; oh shit, they're gone. They were just here." I know I can't get comfortable. I have to constantly hone my craft, take the notes, be nice, and be professional. I've been successful at these so far, and I don't remember getting notes about things I couldn't change or improve— like my body. I recognize that doesn't line up with the stereotype of this industry, and honestly, I might have gotten them, but I truly felt, "This is my body I'm given in the world today." I just didn't have any body insecurity then.

I'm from the South, and I think in Southern black culture, there's a different attitude with size. How I grew up, we didn't have that whole, "You're too big" thing. We had, "Girl, you need to eat something; you're too skinny." So there just wasn't a crack for body insecurity to seep into. And frankly, I liked where my soul lived. I was thick and strong.

I've become more insecure about my body in my later life. Once menopause hit, I felt generally uncomfortable— and I'm all about comfort in clothes, my skin, and flowing through the world. My hormones were all whacked. Because of that, my shape got thicker, which is common. I also gained weight and had a vicious bout with some unpleasant symptoms. My belly was inflamed all the time. I knew I wasn't feeling like me, but not wanting to interrupt my busy schedule, I bought bigger clothes and kept going.

Then, during a photo shoot, the celebrity gave me a note that my outfit did not flatter me. The implication? I reflected poorly on her. I had never received this kind of feedback before. I asked myself, "Is she right about the outfit not flattering me?" I answered, "Yes." Although her comment was curt, it—and my body—got my attention.

Needing to find my way back to feeling normal, to being myself, I sought medical help for my hormones. Though my armor had cracked a little (meaning insecurity about my body existed where none had before), at least I got back to feeling comfortable in my skin.

Years later, I was going along, minding my own business, and backing up another headliner, who I'll refer to as "Art," short for simply "an artist" (gender will not be specified). We'd just finished sound check when Frankie, Art's assistant, walked into the green room. She looked at me with an apologetic expression and said, "Okay, Art wants me to get you in your Bling-two costume." I asked, "Why?" She threw her hands up in an "I don't know" gesture. I then realized that my boss was only calling on me, not the other singers.

Something felt wrong. Frankie and I had been friends for years, and neither of us had any idea what could be happening. This particular award-winning artist had dressed people down before with their cruel streak, but we couldn't figure out why they'd be targeting me right then.

I finished zipping my costume, and we walked into Art's office. There, my boss inspected me, shook their head, and bemoaned, "I don't know what we're going to do."

"What do you mean?" I asked.

Art explained, "You've gained weight. You don't look good in this costume anymore, and these costumes cost me a lot of money."

Art continued to accuse me of gaining weight and ruining their image. I could hear Frankie's and my breathing. Trying to calm my rage and doing my best *not to* say, "You can fuck yourself. I quit. I'm not going to take this from you," I could hear this little voice inside me saying, "You need this job, you want this job, and you enjoy this job. What are you gonna do? What are you going to say?"

I pressed my shoulders back and spoke slowly. "First of all, thank you for letting me know how you feel, but what would you like to *do*?" I stood there, silently waiting for an answer. I could hear this now-not-so-little-voice inside me screaming, "Either fire me, or take the body that I've been given."

Art said they didn't know what to *do* about it because of...this, that, and the other. I interrupted the litany of excuses and again spoke slowly, deliberately, "Okay, we have to perform in three hours. What would you like to *do*?"

I still hoped for a civilized discussion, like talking about how we could make this work for both of us. Instead,

Art kept coming at me sideways, being ugly. Finally, I said, "I don't know what to say. I'm sorry you're not happy."

Then Frankie jumped in: "I have an extra body briefer. Let's try that."

As we left Art's office, I felt myself falling into a hole. Humiliated, I put the little body briefer thing on and marched my happy ass back in there. My boss said, "Oh, that looks really good."

"Thanks," I flatly said and left the room.

Coldcocked! It was like someone hit me in my face. I didn't know what to *do* because my body is what it is. I can't just shave off parts. I fell apart. All my tucked away insecurities flooded me. "I'm not worthy of being here." "I've never been good enough." "I screwed up and it's my fault." "I'm going to be abandoned—thrown out like trash."

Now at this point, I was starting to plunge deeper into that hole. But anger filled me, which was good because when I'm irate, I go into action. I did what I do. I asked myself, is Art *right* about this?

I didn't *think* so, but I don't weigh myself. I went to my friend's house and asked if I looked like I'd gained weight. I needed to be real since part of my job description included not changing my appearance drastically. They said no, but I figured they were probably saying that because they love me.

I decided that I'd take my power back about my body and do what I love to do: reconnect to the appreciation, force, and strength of it through Pilates and yoga. This wasn't oriented towards me trying to lose ten pounds. This was like punching it out, cathartic in that it helped me move that shit through me.

Next, I asked myself, "What can I learn from this?"

Instead of letting the humiliation stay a secret, I shared what happened with a dear friend, who had also worked with my boss. She was furious at Art and hurt by what Art said to me (and you know that misery loves company). My friend said something that helped me find calm space amid the rage and embarrassment: "Remember this is coming from Art's own pain." She reminded me that Art doesn't nourish or possibly even like themself. And for real, that made sense. In spite of that, I was still the one stuck with a sense of wrongness, like my body was bad.

I reached out to a friend from forever ago. She's a mental health practitioner, and I knew she worked with body image stuff. I shared what happened, and she said something pivotal: "You were probably treated as Art treats Art—inside." That was deep. Understanding it that way, I could feel compassion for my boss.

In this process, something else unconscious became conscious. Years ago, I had visited the National Museum of African American History and Culture in D.C. Black women, we have a lot of shame in our DNA from slavery. We were routinely raped, used as breeders, and made to nurse white babies. Our husbands and our own babies were taken away from us. Our skin color determined what level of slave we'd be slotted to, house or field. Deep in my bones, I felt it: *I'm here because of my ancestors, and I have to speak for them. No, I will not be a slave to someone else's expectations of how I should look in my body.*

I had been with Art's show for years at that point. Why they flipped out when they did? Art seems to like to blindside people and then rip them to shreds. I've since discovered that many of us have been through something similar, or even way worse. This multi-award-winning artist has the control and fame, and people want to keep their jobs. Sadly, there are no teeth to human resources in this industry. Therefore, powerful people can run wild sometimes, behaving poorly.

Looking back, I could have easily stayed stuck in that hole, that shame-filled hole—maybe gotten lost there. Before this incident, boundaries had kept me safe. I can trace that back to every single instance where I felt that somebody was coming for me. I was usually the first person to tell them, "You don't have access to that." This one snuck up on me.

****

What pulled me out of the hole was this:

- not letting humiliation silence me
- reaching out for support

- contacting someone who could help me see a broader picture or helpful perspective
- feeling my anger
- doing more of what makes me appreciate my body
- connecting to who I am and what I hold dear
- having a history of strong boundaries that I'm not afraid to stand in. (At this age, I better not be. If I were 25, maybe my boundaries would be different because I hadn't learned how to practice them yet. Once drilled, boundaries feel so good and make life feel pretty safe most of the time.)

****

I still notice the pain that body-shaming incident caused me, and that's mine to nurture. Art doesn't get access to it.

A long time ago, a mentor taught me to stop trying to get rid of something negative I continually felt. When I asked her, "Then what do I do about it?" she said to "invite it along with you." From her, I learned that if I stayed with the feeling and didn't give it power by trying to move away from it, it lost its ability to overwhelm me—instead, fading into simply being *with* me. So, again, I've had to do that.

And my boss? Not surprisingly, Art continues to show up as Art. They're still looking at me sideways a little any time I work with them, but I'm not going to honor it. They can fire me or take the body that I'm giving them.

Note from Alli:

This Storyteller might have had the briefest stay in body dissatisfaction and body shame of all the stories contained in this book. Yet she powerfully felt both. No matter how short of a time someone endures either, the impact can permanently alter a person's life and derail a person's otherwise solid sense of self. With her job potentially depending on it, an impulse-solution could have been to accommodate: change the body to please the boss. This Storyteller instead fixed her issues in a different way—by working through them, deepening her self-awareness.

Although this Storyteller's shaming came from a person in power, we all probably recognize that body insults can happen anywhere and from anyone. Words can wound deeply. And shame tends to stick around when our silence locks it inside us.

Like our Storyteller, using your voice might be a key for conquering you own body dissatisfaction and body shame.

Let Me Pull You Aside

Aaron Flores

AS A FATHER of 10-year-old twins, I hope they never struggle with food or their bodies the way I did. As a professional dietitian, the words that now guide me every day are, "Do no harm." For both my kids and my clients, my wish is that they will deeply know this: what they eat does not make them good or bad, their bodies are amazing at any size, and they can challenge societal values that say anything different. Let's back up though. To know where I am now, we first have to look at where I came from.

It wasn't quite Stepford wives, but close.

I grew up in an affluent, suburban, predominantly white town. Appearance was important and seemed to indicate status. Kids often received a BMW or Mercedes Benz for their first car. I got a Volkswagen Fox.

In high school, I played volleyball. I had above-average skills, but my genetics had dealt me cards that would never allow me to excel in the sport. I wasn't tall, couldn't jump high, and was slightly bigger-around-the-waist than my teammates. No matter how much I trained or worked-out (and I did both a lot), my physique seemed to have an athletic maximum. It refused to look "cut" or get "defined." I got to play during "garbage time," when our team was killing the other team. Otherwise, I sat on the bench.

To help me lose weight and learn "better eating habits," my mom recommended I see a dietitian she'd worked with in the past. Okay. No harm in meeting with her. Maybe she'd help me lose a few pounds. I went along with it.

During the first meeting, that dietitian began teaching me how to count calories and limit my food intake. She directed me to use natural peanut butter only, soak up all the excess oil with a paper towel, and scoop out the insides of my bagels, hollowing them. She prescribed limits for how much of each specific food group I should eat in a day. She assigned me to journal my food 100% of the time. I'd get weighed the next week and each week after that.

Fun times.

I saw her for about three months. I have vivid memories of completing my food journal while parked outside of her high-rise condo. Filling in multiple days at once, I'd furiously write a fictional list of foods I'd eaten while "following" the meal plan she had recommended. I didn't want to get in trouble for blank pages.

This fairly conventional mode of "helping me" to lose weight and eat "healthy" made a lasting impact. I

83

discovered that the focus of traditional weight loss was and is rooted in the shaming of our bodies and behaviors, particularly eating. (Any behavior change rooted in shame is unsustainable.) I also received the clear message that existing in a larger body was only acceptable if I was changing it to a smaller one.

In my 20's, the food-rebel in me ruled my life. For the first time, I lived on my own. Without any restrictions in place, I could finally eat what I wanted, and I did. I'd have pizza at 11 p.m.—not a slice but a whole pizza.

After quitting college, I worked in the tech industry and hated it. I went home with a good paycheck but feeling empty. I craved more meaning in my life.

I didn't have a partner, I had no real direction, and life was getting difficult. I figured my body was the problem. Like, I had a hard time tying my shoes. I thought that if I was smaller, I'd be happier, generally more able, and everything would get better.

One morning, I woke up and said, "I'm going to lose weight." Simple as that. Instead of looking at the real problems in my life, I viewed changing my body as *the fix*.

Years of strict food rules followed. Those dormant edicts awakened. No bagel without scooping. No peanut butter oil. No desserts. No soda. My daily existence became a life of "No," and not just around food either. I started to think that living in a larger body was a "No." No, I wasn't worthy of love, friendship, a career, or connection while in a larger body.

No matter how much weight I lost, I still lived in *that* body. I believed both it, and I, would never be accepted. Feeling uncomfortable in my own skin affected my social life. For example, I wouldn't go play basketball because "shirts vs. skins" concerned me. Which team would I end up on?

I stayed on this path for over three years. I never once called it a *diet*. I told others, and myself, "I'm making healthier choices. This is my new lifestyle." (Total BS, but that's what I said.)

Dieting and losing weight came with mixed experiences. On the one hand, I lived a rigid life, full of rules. Watching my weight was like driving down the road at 100 miles per hour. The path was clear, but I had to be hyper-vigilant. Any deviation would send me careening off the road to certain doom.

On the other hand, I felt exhilarated when people looked at me differently or said, "You look great! You've lost weight." Nobody stared at me when I ate alone in public. I finally blended in. No one seemed to care what I was eating, which was liberating. No one rolled their eyes when I sat next to them on the airplane. People started to flirt with me. A woman randomly gave me her number and card after seeing me with a guy friend at a restaurant. I didn't have to worry about fitting into a booth when eating out, or a seat at a sporting event.

This all felt good.

Despite all the praise, newfound confidence, and freedom to navigate this fat-phobic society with a little bit of thin(ner) privilege, I was completely miserable. I obsessed about food and counted every calorie. Everything went in my food journal. I worked out during my lunch break. I weighed myself two to three times daily. And all this ramped up, especially when my weight loss plateaued.

At this point in my life, I had acquired a vast amount of knowledge about food and dieting, and I still hated my tech job. I started to decipher what kind of work would fit me and feel meaningful. I read that classic book, *What Color is Your Parachute?* which helped me see that I was drawn to working with people, providing a service, and influencing the customer. I already knew I wanted to teach and inspire others to lose weight (and maybe it would further help me with that, too). What career could be a better fit than registered dietitian? I decided to take a huge leap.

In my new profession, I automatically focused on the world of weight loss. I believed that this intervention was the best way to help improve people's health. I knew no other path at that time.

For years, I worked with military veterans. Despite accomplishing important things in their lives—like healing from trauma and successfully assimilating into civilian life—I often watched them beat themselves up because of a number on the scale. This troubled me, but I persisted in working as I'd been trained.

As part of my job, I had to fulfill my continuing education requirements, which meant redundant nutrition lectures for professionals. One totally typical day, I showed up for yet another. Only the presenter said things like, "Most dieters regain weight over time," and, "When we give ourselves unconditional permission to eat, we learn to eat in moderation."

Excuse me?

What?

A life-changer began. I had felt frustrated with my own failed weight-loss attempts. Those vets also struggled with weight loss and experienced anguish as a result of my work. I sensed that I was doing more harm than good. I wanted to do something differently. I wanted to practice differently. Now married with kids, I wanted my whole family to live differently. This nutrition lecturer spoke with compassion and empathy, qualities that truly resonated with me. I picked up the book she co-authored, *Intuitive Eating*.

Filled with humane, non-shaming approaches to nutrition, I saw its potential to help and heal both my clients and me. In a rush of excitement, I emailed this author and presenter, sharing my gratitude. Within hours, she responded and invited me to a supervision group she led each month. I jumped at the opportunity, and for over three years, I attended these sessions. They inspired me to think analytically about my food rules, how I viewed my body, and how I planned to apply non-diet concepts to both my personal life and professional work.

****

I realized I didn't have to live with strict food rules my entire life like I'd thought. My beating-myself-up-over-food could stop. At home, my wife noticed a happier me. I relaxed about feeding the kids, allowing them to build their own relationships with food (not adopt my former relationship with it). We gave them permission to eat whatever they wanted, in any amounts they desired. If they ate only one thing, then that's what they had for dinner. Sometimes, we'd put out dessert with everything at once. They could eat dessert first if they wanted. Our goal was for food to be *a* thing, not the most important thing.

At my job, I *wanted* to proclaim loudly and without hesitation, "Dieting will not improve your health. It does more harm than good. Learning to accept our genetic blueprint is the beginning of changing our relationship with food." However, I feared the effect on my career. A medical community that emphasized thinness as *the* intervention for nearly any chronic medical condition still expected me to prescribe the *whats* and the *how-tos* for weight loss. Yet a person's eating *whys* interested me more.

I could no longer straddle the two opposite paradigms. I took another huge leap.

I now live in the world of weight-inclusivity. I help people make health choices not focused on weight. Intuitive

Eating, Health At Every Size®, and Body Trust® philosophies have profoundly influenced me.

I know how liberating it is to feel at home in my body, no matter what shape or size. I have a relationship with food that's not based in fear or shame, but trust and curiosity. Permission-over-restriction allowed me to be more authentically me. This is who I am. I can't hide it by being thin.

Looking back on my journey, I now recognize the following: my genetics started me off as heavier than my peers, and then all my dieting messed up my natural state. Back when I was bingeing and striving to lose weight, if a professional had looked at my behaviors, without considering my gender or body size, they would've said I had an eating disorder. Because I am male and not emaciated, I flew under the radar. The reality is that people of any size and gender can, and do, get eating disorders.

****

This is the body I have now. I'm good with it, and it's good to me.

I identify as fat. It's a description, not a moral judgment. My life feels purposeful, enjoyable, and connected to others. True health is more than a number on a scale.

I repeatedly witness how a non-diet approach helps many of my clients too.

My children are Intuitive Eaters, meaning they honor their hunger, fullness, and cravings. They are at home in their bodies (so far). I hope that as they get older, they will have gained enough confidence and wisdom to never go on a diet.

I acknowledge that, with the diet culture so prevalent, it's difficult to challenge the idea that "thin bodies are preferred" or "thin is healthier than fat." And even though I would have never believed it back then, I wish that someone would have pulled me aside and said, "Hey Aaron, there is another way!"

So dear reader, let me pull you aside and say this: "There is another way."

It might seem scary to live in a life without diets but the reality is this: it's a very peaceful and very loving relationship with food, which then translates to self and others. Even though this sounds cliché, *when you accept and love your body for what it is, you have permission to take better care of it.*

Note from Alli:

Our Storyteller, Aaron, began trying to lose weight and change his basic genetic build while in his teens. Many of us may have started then too. Food plans and working out are usually the recommendations to win the weight war, yet he did those for years. He ultimately and unconventionally conquered his battles by giving up traditional dieting completely, forming a compassionate relationship with self and food, accepting the influence of genetics, and adopting new methods that served his life instead of diminished it.

You might have reacted to Aaron identifying as "fat." If you did, that's a strong start to noticing the word's power for you. We ALL have judgments (biases) inside us—it's human. And they can keep us stuck too.

A way to begin conquering your own battles with food, weight, and body image is to become more aware of what how you think and feel about the "f" word. What does it mean to you? Just take a breath and notice. Try not to judge yourself, your thoughts, or your feelings. Here's why: if we can face these hidden parts of us with clarity and calmness, we may begin to treat ourselves (and others) with more tolerance and compassion.

There's a social justice movement that focuses on challenging and changing the biases and myths that surround people in larger bodies—The Fat Acceptance Movement. If interested, you can find out more about it in the online article, "8 Things Everyone Should Know about the Fat Acceptance Movement," by Miranda Fotia.[8] Heads-up: if you decide to Google the topic, you'll probably discover that some articles contain strong emotions and perspectives. Look for what helps you, and recognize the pain and oppression involved in the experiences shared.

---

[8] Fotia, *8 Things Everyone Should Know About the Fat Acceptance Movement*, (2018).

It's important to highlight here that certain illnesses (e.g., diagnosed Crohn's, celiac, hemochromatosis, diabetes, etc.) may call for nutritional attention. This story was not about that. If you have questions about a non-diet approach or a chronic disorder that can include dietary recommendations, please consult with a professional; a Registered Dietitian/Registered Dietitian Nutritionist who is trained in Intuitive Eating and Health At Every Size® (HAES®) principles can offer a potentially different, valuable perspective for you to consider. Both have been included in the Resources section of this book. Each honors a non-diet approach and encourages people of all sizes to adopt lifestyles that can benefit mental and physical health.

I Am That Girl

Veronica Garcia

AT THE AGE of four, I witnessed someone shooting at my father as he ran. This was over a parking spot. In my neighborhood where I grew up, the gangs owned the streets. We were very poor. Both my parents worked full time, and then some, to make ends meet. Because of this, we five kids mostly raised ourselves.

I am *that girl*. The one who has to learn things the hard way. The lesson has got to be in my face, and I usually have to lose sleep wondering, "Why am I in this place?" Otherwise, good chance I'll repeat the behavior again and again.

Here's what I mean. In the 9th and 10th grades, I ditched, did drugs, and partied instead of being in school. For that year and a half, I forged my parents' names on my horrible report cards. I ended up having to repeat the 10th grade in a remedial class.

One day, I looked around at my classmates in remedial. I noticed the majority showed no signs of wanting to change or to stop causing trouble. I thought, "Why am I doing this to myself? I don't want to go where they're probably going in life. Shape up, Veronica!"

I then did everything I could to get back to where I thought I belonged—adding classes, taking extra ones, and making up those I failed. I challenged myself by taking AP (Advanced Placement) Economics with a teacher who was known for both her toughness and for failing people. I got a good grade, which I took as a sign—I had worked myself closer to my own right track.

Back in my childhood, no one taught me about communication and feelings, the birds and the bees, or anything in between. What I figured out, the streets taught me. The following principles guided me during the first few decades of my life:

- Women should be sexy, attract men, and make babies.

- Always "Be unfuckable with." That meant show no weaknesses, suck it up, never ask for help, and don't let anyone see you cry.

That need to be unshakable matched something my parents communicated. "We came from Mexico, and we had to battle this, and we had to do that, and if you're going to sit there and let that beat you, you are the one who loses."

Not wanting to lose, when I felt emotions, I found my ways to deal with them: playing sports, fighting... and eating. As a kid, I played a lot of sports in the streets with the guys. Physical activity was probably my healthiest coping strategy, and I kept it up into adulthood. Once I had my own kids, though, I didn't have the time to do any organized athletics. All sports went away.

Fighting as a way to deal with emotions worked well for me in childhood. As an adult, it did not. It once got me, at least 20 girls, and a handful of guys detained outside a club, wrists tie-wrap handcuffed behind our backs. I spent that long holiday weekend in jail—another *in my face* lesson.

That left eating. My family used food to soothe each other. Not surprisingly, I picked up the habit, too. Besides, eating fit in easily between all the things a single mother has to do.

Though I did not eat a lot at one sitting, I ate often. If I felt stressed, I ate. If I felt sad or happy, I ate. If someone visited, we ate together. Over and over, I ate and we ate. In my culture, it's rude if we don't offer food or eat with our guests.

After my second child, I remember watching this woman who was wearing a hot dress I liked. I thought, "She could look really good if she didn't have that belly sticking out." I went and found the same dress at the mall, tried it on, and crap! I had the same belly sticking out.

My formerly thin frame had grown. I had always had large breasts, but never shapely thighs or a tummy.

Since straighter figures were in fashion and desirable at the time, I started to diet to shed some pounds. I also bought a used treadmill. Any chance I could, I ran and did push-ups and sit-ups.

When I finally exercised and dieted enough to fit into my pants with nothing hanging out—no muffin top—I'd feel good. Then I'd relax and ditch the diet. The weight would come back on, I'd think, "Shit, I did it again!" and then start over. For about ten years, I did this routine.

I got really skinny once. It was that time when straight frames, big boobs, and showing a midriff were "in." Someone said, "You kinda look dead. You lost your cheeks." Looking dead was obviously not sexy.

When I reflect back, my dieting and exercising kept me company. They filled my time, and maybe took the place of romantic relationships. I rarely dated; I felt terrified of it. However, as my teen children transitioned into young adults, thoughts of "I'm going to be alone for the rest of my life" kept me up at night. I knew I needed to "get back out there," try to date, and (hopefully) marry someday.

My first night out, I sat at a table near the dance floor in an outfit that I thought camouflaged all my flaws. I wore silver stretch pants to eliminate the cupcake tummy roll, a black top, tall heels. I compared myself to sexy-looking, thin women ten years younger. I watched men buy them drinks. My beer? I bought it for myself.

There I was, in the middle of a sea of men. I felt unworthy of love. I knew I didn't want to have any more babies with anyone, which made me feel guilty because I was raised to believe that moms are supposed to be unselfish and women are supposed to have babies. At that moment, I believed that I had failed—as a mom, as a woman, and at being attractive. I felt like a loser and left.

Around this same time, someone else's misfortune changed my life in a good way. While working at a health clinic, one of our therapists came in crying. Her husband had cheated on her, had an affair. As she shared her pain with me, she questioned how he could love her if she didn't love herself.

Love yourself. That was a new concept to me.

I did a quick assessment: I did not love myself. I was not kind or compassionate to myself the way I was to others. I had changed the look of my body over and over again, trying to fit some trendy concept of "desirable" or "sexy." I had only defined myself by a few things. I knew I could leave a relationship and support my children on my own. I also took pride in knowing that nobody told me what to do, that I had not joined any gangs, and that no man ever controlled me. Yet I constantly compared myself to everyone else, and I constantly fell short.

I decided to break the street rule about not asking anyone for help. Through a co-worker, I'd learned that counselors couldn't tell anyone (for the most part) what happened in a session. If no one would know what I said, it would be okay to try therapy. I had to learn who I was. I had to find me—keep what I liked and change what I didn't, *but only for me.*

Here's what I discovered.

****

My negative self-talk had to change.

I started paying attention to what was in my mind and challenging the thoughts. *Is that true? What are the facts?* When my negative self-talk was accurate, I'd have to do something to change it. When the thought was not true, I'd remind myself, "It's just a thought, just energy going through me. It's not real." The more I did this, the more I found myself thinking things like, "I'm smart, I look pretty good, and I do a good job being a parent." I'd also challenge and reinforce those positive thoughts with—*Is that true? What are the facts?*

I had to figure out what truly made me happy.

I did this mostly by making mistakes, but I paid attention, which eventually carved a clear path.

I had to accept "I am who I am, and am not."

I could not be or look like someone else, so I had to stop comparing myself to others. To give an example, I'd see a person at the mall and think, "She's got a good shape." I'd notice the thought and then think something, *anything,* nice about my shape. That would make the comparison thought go away.

I had to ask myself, "Do I need to look like everyone else or follow trends?"

No, I didn't. Being different is okay. I started accentuating my curves in a classic way instead of hiding them. My style of dressing finally fit who I was (and am). It said, "This is me, and that's it."

The hardest part was learning to be alone and not feel like a loser.

It took a six-month process of writing down what I was thinking. Based on my therapist's homework, I would sit in a room, alone, with no television or radio on. She told me to breathe deeply and slowly and write down my thoughts. The minute my thoughts felt "too bad" to "sit with it," I turned on the television, as my therapist had instructed. Later, I'd read what I wrote and then challenge the critical thoughts. I remember asking myself, "Is it true? Am I a loser?" I answered, "I can't be a loser if I support my kids on my own, if I have good kids, a good family, and good friends."

The longer I did this, the less horrible I felt. Gradually, I began looking forward to having alone time and then to appreciating being alone.

Change took a few years of making more conscious, mindful choices based on, "What do I want since I'm going to own the consequences?"

****

I now love myself. Yes, I know that's a big word, but I see loving oneself as liking, being kind to, and accepting the many parts of self, inside and outside—like how you would treat someone you love.

At forty-five, I have four grandbabies. The thought of being able to teach them to love themselves makes my hard lessons worth it. My life feels full and enjoyable. I value sharing it with my two kids and their kids.

I also love my curvy body. It does wonderful things all on its own, with no diets or improvements required. It carried those two kids. It tells me if I'm not being good to it, and when it does, I listen. It's aging, which is making me more comfortable in my skin than I have ever been. It's a beautiful process.

Exercise is no longer about looks or flattening muffin tops. I box, hike, walk, and do other activities to *feel good*. Alive. Activity helps me physically express myself and get my emotions out. Hikes with great company, conversation, and scenery are my favorite.

I don't diet anymore. I don't like feeling hungry. I eat to feel good, meaning that I have a steady source of energy that informs my moods. I enjoy my food and drinks, which also gives me a sense of satisfaction.

I stopped eating to soothe emotions. Instead, I reach out to friends, volunteer for cool projects, research stuff that interests me, take random classes because I love learning, babysit my grand-delicious-babies, and travel alone. I create adventures and appreciate the moments of quiet.

I no longer offer to eat with guests out of obligation. I appreciate someone visiting. I thank them for that, which is enough.

I still have not mastered dating or gotten married, but I'm okay with that. I truly am. I have this one life. I plan on enjoying it with peace of mind. Comparing myself to others, changing my body, and following trends set by anyone but me are OUT of my life. Self-love is IN, even though it takes work (like, every day) to get there.

Note from Alli:

In this story, Veronica used food for coping, connection, and company. Instead of continuing her weight-loss/weight-gain routine, she allowed her ability to "learn things the hard way" to help her find her methods for conquering her issues. Her unorthodox solutions to her problems led to more fulfilling ways of living.

This story also spotlights resourcefulness. Whether we are taught how-tos or are left to self-discovery, we find our coping methods. And in trying to take care of ourselves, sometimes we do things that both hurt AND help us, like emotional eating or this Storyteller's fighting.

Instead of judging yourself as having "poor" or "bad" coping strategies, try congratulating your inner resourcefulness for being so wise. You knew you needed help, and you made that happen. If you now notice that your coping mechanism isn't serving you how you want it to, seek new ways that might enhance your life. As Veronica showed us, experimenting with coping skills can help you to live more of a life you want—while also changing your food and body image struggles into strengths.

What a Trip!

Anonymous

MY PRAYERS FOR a Huckleberry-friend to accompany me on adventures were answered.

Whether finances or not having a partner to roam with had stopped me, I hadn't been able to make my dream of international travel happen. That is, until about a year into dating my now-wife. She said she wanted to share her childhood memories with me, which both touched me and meant a trip to Germany!

Out-of-my-mind excited, I spent a month trying to learn to speak German. We figured out which parts of the country were most important for us to visit. We coordinated staying with a good friend stationed in the military there, which fit our budget (free!). And since she was gay (like us), we knew we could relax and be ourselves around her. Double win.

Seat back upright, buckled in, and ready to take off, the guy loading the luggage punched a hole in the plane.

Bummer. A second canceled flight and fourteen hours later, we arrived tousled, still excited, and ravenous. We headed for the closest and fastest source of food we could locate: McDonalds.

There, I scanned the menu, which to my surprise was written in English. Finding no "healthy" options I could eat, I shrunk back from the counter, slowly walked away, and burst into tears.

Admittedly, this was not a normal reaction. At the time, I was in the throes of orthorexia (which means basically that the perceived need for *pure, clean,* or *healthy* eating takes over a person's diet and life). It had been hours since any snack or meal, and undeniably, I felt hungry. However, I couldn't eat anything "not allowed." I know this might sound extreme, but food combinations and certain foods *not* on my health-optimizing food plan seemed threatening to me, poisonous.

My strictness about eating an exclusively "healthy" diet started years before our trip. A bout of viral mononucleosis had left me with a lack of energy, digestive discomfort, and an element of feeling crappy all the time. Because my medical doctor's advice hadn't helped improve those issues, I started concentrating on my nutrition to hopefully fix the situation. As Hippocrates said, "Let food be thy medicine and medicine be thy food," and I'm a proactive girl.

As an avid reader, I learned what I thought was everything about nutrition. I particularly focused on a popular healthy lifestyle plan that purported to heal ailments through proper food combinations and eliminations. With vigor and hope, I applied my dietary knowledge, and each time I'd start to feel *less* crappy, a period of feeling *even crappier* would then follow. Since I assumed every decline was because I hadn't been strict enough with my nutrition, I'd double down on getting it *perfect.*

Somewhere during this pursuit of health, my diet turned into an obsession. No one noticed it was problematic; the opposite happened. My friends complimented my nutritional knowledge, food choices, and thin appearance. They said they could "never have my discipline."

They didn't know that I absolutely *had* to eat correctly. When I questioned if a food was healthy enough or a food combination good enough, I opted to not consume it, just in case. Whole food groups vanished, and nutrition labels controlled my choices. No hydrogenated oil, no preservatives, and dairy went out the window. The more reading I did, the more stringent I became about whole-foods-only (plant foods, nothing processed or refined).

So fast food, even if on German soil? *Hell no.*

That moment began two weeks of intense fear for me, which often translated into being difficult to be around. "Healthy" food had become synonymous with personal safety, and in a foreign country, I had no control. I had to eat in restaurants where I didn't plan the menu and I couldn't read food labels because they were written in

German. All these factors made eating scary. So for 14 days, I snipped, "No, I cannot eat that particular combination of food," "No, that is not an allowed food," and "I don't know the ingredients. No, I will not eat that."

On the other hand, my then-girlfriend and our friend *just ate*. As they gobbled their pizza *with* cheese (a combination not allowed!), they rolled their eyes at my food-righteousness. (Thinking back, I might have rolled my eyes at it, too. My healthy eating-obsession was judgmental and obnoxious.)

During our stay, our poor friend had repeatedly gotten caught in my food tantrums and my partner's exasperation with me. I remember her saying as we packed to leave, "You guys brought all that emotional crap with you and I'm glad to see you go."

Ouch.

When I arrived home, I plopped our vacation experience in the middle of my therapist's office. I had been seeing her for a while for completely non-food related issues. She just happened to have a specialty in eating disorders.

I shared that famous German landmarks—from castles to salt mines—paled in comparison to the redeeming food stops I longed for: the little cafes that offered wholesome, natural, home-cooked, *safe* foods I could properly combine. I told her that I thought my girlfriend "should have been more understanding about my diet exceptions." I complained that she "should want to take better care of herself."

Filled with assuredness, I waited for my therapist to agree. She instead told me, "Your girlfriend is a grown adult. What are you going to do *for you*? Starving yourself isn't a great way to take care of yourself. Your girlfriend's at least eating, even if it's what you consider horrible food." She explained how harmful restricting food intake was for my heart, especially given how much I was training in martial arts every day, which she advised me to stop.

WHAAAT?

We saw different problems. How could attention on health be a bad thing? Ever?! Besides, she knew I'd been into this lifestyle thing since before I started seeing her. I thought she was overreacting.

Then suddenly, yet another issue materialized— migraine headaches. And of course, the prescription migraine medication from my doctor didn't help. I wondered why I was falling apart when I was working so damn hard to be healthy. (I later learned that with my strange eating habits, over-exercising, and elimination of protein, it would have been a wonder if I *didn't* get migraines.)

Determined, but at a loss for solutions, I explored Eastern medicine. My Chinese medicine practitioner explained that the process of healing would take time, and that treatment would include acupuncture, Chinese herbs, and work on the whole body. I agreed to all of it because, at this point, why not?

While following her instructions, my world began to change in a positive way. After about four months, the headaches decreased while digestion and energy improved. As my body became more balanced, so did my emotions and thinking. I remember waking up one day and realizing it felt entirely different to be in my own mind—as if clouds had moved and unblocked a blue sky. I could see possibilities where none had existed before: maybe I can add bananas on my Grape-Nuts and the world won't end.

Though my therapist was great, I believe I could have been in therapy years longer if I hadn't done the Chinese medicine too. After just a few months, I stopped dismissing the therapist's suggestions to "try a certain food" or "go ahead and eat until you're satisfied." Instead, I took a deep breath and explored my options.

Years after I healed, I went on to become a licensed acupuncturist and let me explain what happened. The acupuncture regulated my nervous system, giving me a more balanced place from which to operate.

Don't get me wrong, the process of restoring balance was not easy, but week after week, I plodded along. Luckily, I had the support of my partner. Her good friend in college and then another in the military had both had eating disorders, so she knew how to be patient and understanding around intense food angst. I remember her holding my hand as I wept, trying to eat black beans and rice. (Why?

Imagine being forced to eat a poisonous scorpion tail or lick a live virus. That's how consuming black beans and rice felt for me—and probably for others who experience orthorexia too).

I knew I was on my way to wellness when one day, after I had gone to a CPR class for my job, I went to Subway. I ate the whole sandwich and a bag of chips, and I did it all by myself. It felt good not to be hungry.

To have a life I wanted—balanced, full, loving, and *actually* healthy—I had to do work. Here's what I think is important to share.

****

Be committed.

You have to show up to whatever help you have committed to, even though there probably won't be immediate results. If you want to get to the source of the problem and not just put a bandage on it, it's not going to be better today. It's going to take several tomorrows.

Be thoughtful about who you choose to help you.

Consider *your* belief systems and choose someone in alignment with your worldview, not your issue's or illness's view. There are many options out there. Eastern medicine will be for some but not for others.

Choosing acupuncture honored both the rebel and intellectual parts of me. People raised their eyebrows, but it was a counterculture that had thousands of years of evidence to support it. I liked both.

Vet your helpers; not all professionals are trained in eating issues.

When my doctor and I talked about my eating disorder, he prescribed a glass of red wine before every meal. This advice was ridiculous and not scientifically founded. Do you know what red wine can trigger? A migraine!

Another example is that many contemporary Chinese medicine practitioners, naturopaths, and other holistic providers encourage the elimination of foods for various reasons. Had I chosen one of those practitioners, I would have gotten physically and mentally sicker. I'm grateful I found a practitioner who knew better.

Be careful what you believe.

There is plenty of erroneous, extreme diet and health information published. One of the most respected and utilized nutritional plans at the time started all the food problems for me. In fact, it's still marketed as a way to optimal health.

Check yourself.

If you are committed to eating healthy, and you look around and see everyone else happy but you're not, you will probably benefit by doing things differently.

Also, it can feel confusing if you're getting uncomfortable symptoms after you eat. A healthy body is supposed to be able to digest and use a wide variety of foods.

If yours isn't doing that, you might need more balance and support.

****

I usually consider my tendencies towards perfectionism, getting things correct, and my determination to be good personality traits. Yet during my healthy eating obsession, I had gone to the extreme. There's a fine line between perseverance and stubbornness, as well as between focus and obsession.

Since recovering from the grip of my "healthy" eating obsession, I go on trips and enjoy them. We most recently visited Panama where we had a fantastic time! Amidst seeing a rainforest, making friends, learning history, watching ships in the Canal, eating a variety of exotic and delicious cuisine, and trying to speak Spanish, my wife and I laughed together a lot (sometimes at me and my clumsy Spanish).

Originally, I tried to solve feeling unwell through improving my diet. This, unto itself, is not a bad thing. I went too far and ended up causing (or at least exacerbating) legit health issues, obsessive-thinking, and relationship problems.

It's still a trip to me that something that starts well-intended can end so not well. Please be suspicious of any dietary pursuit of health that distances you from your loved ones, deprives you of life experiences, or ruins a dream vacation.

Note from Alli:

Like many people, this Storyteller strived for healthy eating (not weight loss) that would make her feel better. It wasn't working, and a common solution to the perceived problem of not eating healthy enough or clean enough is to eat stricter. She did that—and fell into orthorexia. As her narrative shows, a healthy-food obsession damaged her quality of life and relationships, her personality changed to more judgmental, and she encountered maladies likely caused from her strict regimen. To revive her nutrition and overcome her problems, she enlisted non-mainstream, individualized approaches, which resulted in life-enriching realizations and practices.

This story demonstrates that orthorexia can seem like anorexia nervosa because of rigid rules and typical reduction in caloric intake. But a person with orthorexic tendencies focuses more on health and less on losing weight. If a person focuses on both, they probably lean towards anorexia.

As you can see throughout this book, there are fine lines between the different food and body image struggles and diagnoses. At this time, orthorexia is not an official clinical eating disorder—yet. Whether we call something an eating disorder or disordered eating, either can disrupt a person's thinking, emotions, personality, relationships, health, and quality of life.

Lastly—and this may sound counterintuitive—a common and unintended consequence of **any** restrictive, limited diet can be medical malnutrition (which is the opposite of healthy). This can happen to a person of any size or weight. Such cases can require medical monitoring (for safety) and can bring about symptoms of unwellness (people can *appear* hypochondriacal). If you might be at risk for malnutrition from an imbalanced diet, please consider seeing a professional for an evaluation and potential help.

TSA Confiscated My Fake Butter Spray

Aurora Miceli

PICTURE THIS...IT'S the late 1990s in small-town Indiana. The low-fat/no-fat food fad is as popular as Tickle Me Elmo at Christmas. I mean, if you don't eat fat, you can't get fat, right? Luckily, we have learned much more about nutrition in the decades since. But back then, fat-free devil's food SnackWell's cookies were *life*.

I was in high school at the time playing varsity basketball. Our uniform jerseys were numbered from ten up to 40. The sizes grew as the numbers did. I was #11. To stay in that same jersey for four years—so I didn't have to openly admit to simply growing—I joined in the unhealthy relationship with food that had swept the nation.

I still get ghost pains just thinking about the fat-free, gut-wrenching potato chips we ate that were made with Olestra. If you're too young to remember, they literally came with a warning label: "may cause abdominal cramping and loose stools." I once had to help a friend out of her bathtub because of both. (It wasn't her finest moment.) For so many of us, everything moved right through because, while the molecule Olestra tasted like regular fat, our intestines had no idea what to do with it.

I was also a vegetarian and had been since elementary school—so I was eating a tremendous amount of carbohydrates ("simple" carbohydrates, as we call them today). In a whole day, I'd eat nothing but puffed cereal and pretzels. I needed them all the time because they were as filling as eating air. Open up and take a swallow.

Starvation, or at least extreme dietary restriction, was the name of my game. It was part of the trend; everyone was doing it. I made up my own diet program: the five-and-fit diet. (No Internet existed then, and we couldn't afford any real diet programs.) I could eat five different items throughout the day. "Let's see. I've had my puffed cereal, pretzels, a SnackWell's. Two more things, what can I eat?" Talk about a lack of variety! It was a good thing that I Can't Believe It's Not Butter! fat-free spray butter didn't count because it was a condiment. That spray stayed closer to me than a new Boyz II Men single. It made me feel safe. Instead of having self-awareness that something was strange about taking a bottle of fake butter on a plane, I was furious when the newly founded TSA confiscated it.

Looking back, here's how I think this all rolled together. I had been dealing with physical and sexual abuse by a stepparent that had begun around 4th grade and then

115

continued until after high school. My mom was married to the guy, so I hadn't wanted to hurt her feelings or cause a problem for her. He had also groomed me to keep quiet. My sister, a decade older than me, had already moved out by the time it began, and it was just me living in the same house with someone violent.

In junior high, I was still a good girl who hung out at the mall. Then during high school, I started lashing out at school against teachers and coaches. I began engaging in risky behavior (staying out late or not coming home, drinking, boys—things you wouldn't want your own kids doing). In my tight food restrictions, I found the feeling of safety that I was lacking. My five-and-fit diet created a sort of unbending formula I could rely on and trust, and that seemed to calm me while so much else felt ablaze. Dieting made me feel in control of myself.

To get away from the abuser, I chose a college two states away. When I left, I took my books and those restrictive, rigid eating habits right along with me. I went to a Catholic university (of course—I'm Italian). Living in an all-girl's residence hall was like living in the epicenter of a women's fiction novel. We shared class notes, clothes, secrets, and diet tips. This is when I added purging to my repertoire. We'd go out on a Friday night and think nothing of heading right into the bathroom when we got back to the dorm if we felt we ate or drank too much. For lack of a better term, it was essentially a puke party. We'd take turns, discussing it afterward like a play-by-play commentator. Our attitudes and behaviors were contagious amidst each other, a sort of bonding in sisterhood.

One winter break, I travelled to Orange County with my college friend. The weather there was *beautiful!* She lived on 12 acres in a fancy area. We drove down, crossed the border, and partied in Mexico. I fell in love with Southern California.

At 20 years old, I decided I needed to completely change my whole situation. After returning home, I packed my bags for "SoCal" and made plans to live with someone in San Diego. When those plans fell through, I suddenly realized: "Wait! LA is there, right?"

I arrived in the famed City of Angels with almost nothing. I'd always been a good planner, but it took me a little while to find my way because I was alone in a foreign land.

Immediately, I bought a clunker car, lived in it for the first six weeks, and showered at a gym where I could afford a membership. I moved in with the guy (not romantically) who had sold me my car insurance. He was strange. He once left his girlfriend on the side of the road, stranded. He told me he wanted to test her crisis management skills.

Living with him did not feel secure.

I then moved in with someone a friend knew. After a few months there, I came home to a barricade. The FBI had raided the house because of illegal gambling. Still, I stayed, until one day, I grabbed a couple brownies and left to hang out at a friend's house. No one told me they were laced with marijuana, and paranoia filled me. I screamed at people to call the cops because I was going to be killed. Such a horrible experience, mostly because I could not tolerate feeling out of control or threatened. I drew the line there and moved out.

Eventually, I found a stable living situation, got myself enrolled in school, obtained a reliable job, and made new friends (who didn't test people's crisis skills or lace brownies with drugs). Most importantly, I finally felt safe enough to tell my family about the abuse I had endured.

I found out that my mom was thinking about leaving her husband. I believed he was an alcoholic, and I wanted her to be done with him. Hoping it would help her decision, I felt I could finally say it, "Oh, well, by the way…" By then, I had already told my sister, who had received me with love and support. But telling Mom? That was nerve-wracking for me.

She listened, apologized, and didn't defend him. Mom must have felt safe enough to leave. All of us were out.

That was a real game changer for me—dealing with the trauma. I was able to release a lot of the fear, hate, and doubts I had about myself. What remained has required attention at times throughout the years.

With all the warped food stuff I did, and for as long as I did it, I never got an eating disorder. Once I was presented with enough space and safety to stop those behaviors, I did so, and easily. I didn't even notice I was eating in a healthier way. It felt as natural as the coastline I witnessed for the first time when I arrived in LA. I didn't miss or think about any of it, not the five-and-fit diet, not the puking, and not even my beloved I Can't Believe It's Not Butter! spray. I simply moved onward and forward.

I'm still a vegetarian. That was something I committed to early on. It's a core part of my values, and my volunteerism reflects it. I'm always donating time to local animal shelters.

Despite those years of a live-to-eat focus, I've discovered that I'm more of an eat-to-live person. I can enjoy eating, but I'm not a foodie. I grew up low income. That showed me I could probably eat simple, repetitive food and be fine with it. But still, when someone cooks something tasty? Then I'm a "this is delicious, can I have seconds?" person.

I'm a natural athlete and have always played sports. Part of that gym membership those first few weeks in California? I need to be active, it's part of my being. Though it probably helps me to feel like "me" in my body, activity has never been about weight. I am strong and like to feel strong.

I've found the joy of real butter. I eat enough of it to make a pastry chef proud.

****

Dieting lost its hold on me years ago and I can proudly say, as a vivacious 35-year-old ER nurse, I have never felt better, safer, or more connected to life and with people.

With hindsight, I have the wisdom to see how my restrictive eating and purging helped give me order and structure within chaos. For many years, I couldn't speak my way to safety. So I had to find a way there on my own. Clearing up the trauma helped to clear up my eating stuff.

****

If you are doing weight management behaviors that would be deemed "unhealthy" in the long run, maybe wonder: "Besides for weight, why am I doing this?" It's a hard question, and I'm pretty sure that back then, I would have answered without a full picture: "It's JUST to manage my weight." But maybe not. And maybe this question helps someone reading this.

And now, this brings me to Mister Rogers. You know how he says to look for a helper in a time of crisis? That ended up being my sister, before I was able to tell my mom that difficult information. With every crisis (housing, money, breakups), there has always been a helper I could find. If you are in crisis, look for a helper. It might be you.

Note from Alli:

This Storyteller, Aurora, enlisted food restriction and purging to help her control her weight. She unexpectedly conquered all three—restriction, purging, and weight management—in unpredicted ways: by dealing with her trauma, by organizing some of the danger and chaos in her life, and by getting herself safe from harm. Could your eating issues be serving to soothe or distract you from something painful that needs your attention?

Aurora does not identify with having had an eating disorder. And with her ease of stopping the behaviors and resuming regular eating, that makes sense to me. Confusing, huh?

If you're wondering whether you might have an issue more serious than originally thought, here is a simple, informal experiment that can help you assess your own status. Think of any food or weight-related practices you have, and try not doing those practices for a few hours, a day, a week—kind of like you can test if you might have an issue with alcohol when you try NOT drinking. If you restrict, try eating. If you purge, try keeping your food inside you. If you exercise to compensate for what you ate, try skipping the workout. You'll probably get a sense of how powerful NOT doing your behavior feels to you. There's support out there, no matter what you discover.

"Puke parties" as weight-control come with far-reaching risks. Making yourself throw up can disrupt your metabolism and bring on symptoms of dehydration, ranging from mild to severe. Teeth enamel may become weakened or eroded from repeated vomiting (new teeth=expensive). Your internal balance (e.g., electrolytes) can become dangerously unbalanced. Severe malnutrition can happen, which in addition to causing medical problems, usually makes you look unwell. You can also unexpectedly experience heart problems that can be deadly. And...so many more.

For information about risks of purging, you may appreciate reading the online scholarly journal article, "The Medical Complications Associated with Purging," by Forney and colleagues.[9] But if you find yourself searching the Internet instead (as so many of us do), you'll probably discover that titles will often include the words "bulimia" or "eating disorders." Please don't let the thought of "I don't have either" limit your results. Information empowers.

No one can predict how a body will react to forced vomiting, and there is no formula for how often, much, or long one can do it before consequences happen. These built-in threats from nature remind us that our bodies do not consider any form of purging to be a viable option for weight maintenance or loss.

I need to say something here about trauma, which can be viewed as a deeply distressing life event. Again, no one can predict how a body or mind will react to having experienced it. Trauma is a huge topic, and there are treatments for it. Bessell van der Kolk, M.D., is a pioneer and expert in the field. His book, *The Body Keeps the Score: Brain, Mind, and Body in the Healing of Trauma*[10] could be helpful to read.

---

[9] Forney et al., *The Medical Complications Associated with Purging*, (2016).
[10] van der Kolk, *The Body Keeps the Score: Brain, Mind, and Body in the Healing of Trauma*, (2014).

If you have experienced trauma, finding your ways of working through it and getting safer might offer you a different, preferred tomorrow.

Awakening

Beau-Haim Harang

BEING A MORTICIAN and funeral director has showed me I have a huge talent for makeup colors. I repeatedly heard, "Oh wow! My mother has never looked this good!" as Mum lay there, lifeless but looking red-carpet-ready.

These kinds of compliments propelled me to pursue a career as a makeup artist for "the living." After my formal training, I auditioned for a huge brand that was launching a nationwide makeup artist program. Competing against thousands, I placed in the top 12. The ensuing exposure and relationships catapulted me into a career as a celebrity makeup artist.

The fashion and beauty world became my home. Major events such as the Oscars®,[11] Young Hollywood Awards, and fashion shows for Vera Wang and Carolina

---

[11] The Oscars® is a registered trademark of the Academy of Motion Picture Arts and Sciences.

Herrera became commonplace for me. After that, I had three other high-powered jobs and excelled at all of them. With the advanced skills needed for professional success, you'd think I'd have mastered basic, personal self-care—but I hadn't.

For more than two decades, I didn't feed myself enough, exercised too much, binged, and purged. I collapsed from weakness countless times, and was hospitalized at ages 18, 24, 27, and 30.

I come from a long line of high achievers; perfectionism was natural. Lawyers on my father's side, doctors on my mother's, and an uncle who was ambassador of a Central American country. There I was, a creative artist born into this academic/political family, and a Jew in a Catholic school to boot. I felt I didn't fit in. I didn't shine like everybody else, especially my family members.

So at ten years old, when my favorite aunt told me I could be in her wedding if I lost ten pounds, I happily agreed. (This was a well-intended, misguided attempt at protecting me from family "obesity.") To me, this meant that in just a few pounds, I'd finally *feel* accepted.

This perfectionist lost 20, was praised, and made it into the wedding. But nothing else changed. I didn't understand. I figured I must have missed something. Here's where a driving force set in: if I could just get my body *right*, I'd be good enough, I'd feel accepted, and I'd feel comfortable inside instead of *so uncomfortable*. Moving forward, I pursued this with gusto.

The cycles—undereating and over-exercising, which led to losing control and bingeing, which led to trying to fix the binge by purging—were vicious. But I could not stop the cycles or change the thoughts and behaviors that accompanied them. At the same time, I delusionally believed that I was in control. I had gotten an eating disorder.

From age 10 to 32, professionals diagnosed me with various illnesses: bulimia nervosa, anorexia nervosa, binge-eating disorder, depression, and even lymphoma (cancer). I recognized each diagnosis was *supposed* to be a big deal. A two-week "forced stabilization" in the hospital was certainly harsh consequence of my cycles. However, I couldn't see the seriousness of *any* of the diagnoses (except the cancer).

Repeatedly, I'd collapse from lack of nutrients and weakness. But even if I tried the eating disorder treatment programs that hospitals or friends would recommend, I found that as a male, treatment wasn't fitting. One place refused me after a lengthy intake because my gayness might provoke or influence the girls on the unit... what?! When I was not rejected for being male, gay, too sick, or too thin, I'd get out of the program and immediately return to my cycles. Whether it was bad treatment or I wasn't ready, I'm not sure. But I'd keep moving in life—accomplishing professionally while still seeking acceptance and a sense of internal "comfortableness."

My turning point happened in 2010. Extremely exhausted from eating little to nothing, over-exercising, lying, and self-sabotaging, I had traveled to Dallas to attend a huge art exhibit with my friend, Michel, a fellow art lover. Throughout the weekend, I hid food, avoided eating with excuses (e.g., "I already ate"), and woke up super early to exercise while he slept.

As usual, people complimented me on my ever-changing look and style. I posed with the artists for the paparazzi. The weekend seemed normal: *until it didn't*.

Driving back to his place after an event, a strange, stagnant quiet filled the car. When we arrived, his words sliced through the silence. "You have a deeply bad problem. You're sick."

I knew he was not referring to my recent remission from cancer, but I didn't understand. "What are you talking about?"

He replied with a loving intensity, "I don't have to explain. I saw this whole week."

My heart dropped. "What did you see?"

He said, "I see someone who is literally starving himself, over-exercising, and overcompensating for what he is missing."

Panic filled my body. I couldn't lose the only friend I had left. So many people had mysteriously fallen away from me, so he was it. Desperate to remain connected, I asked, "Can you help me through this?" He said, "I'm incapable. I'm not licensed, and the type of help that you need is very deep. Unfortunately, I cannot be friends with you until you get the help that you need, and you recognize how sick your actions are." And he left.

I turned off the engine, looked up at the closed garage he disappeared into, and completely lost my shit. My eyes were so filled with tears I was unable to see. As I wiped them, sobbing uncontrollably, I couldn't stop thinking about it. Here's what my disorder heard my friend say: "Beau, you are weak, emotional, and not man enough." *This* was my interpretation of his heartfelt wake-up plea, which shows how your mind turns to mush from starvation. When I got my shit together enough to drive away, the worry crippled me: who else would he tell? I was already so alone.

By mid-afternoon the next day, I'd decided I needed help, but I didn't know who to call or what to do. Pure disgust started to unfold over how long I had allowed the disorder to take over my life. I started to cry uncontrollably again.

Suddenly, my cell phone rang. It was my sister calling. Though not completely close during these years, she could always connect with me and help me feel safe and cared for in times of despair. Without hesitation, I answered. My voice trembled as I held back my breakdown. "Hello?"

She always started our phone calls with "Hey, it's me." I paused, and she quickly responded, "You okay?" Once again, I remained silent. Finally, she said, "Beau?" I could no longer hold back what I had done to myself—once again.

I remember it vividly. I said, "I can't live this way. I am tired."

She responded without hesitation, "Pack your bag and head over to Aunt Jew's house. You need to be in a safe place." She gave me instructions to be there within one hour. She happened to be a therapist specializing in eating disorders. Her clear directions comforted me.

Bags filled and on the way to my aunt's home, I began to think about how I was going to approach this with my sister and mum. This wouldn't be my first time "going to school" to be taught my own needs, emotionally and nutritionally. But when I arrived at my aunt's, there was almost no discussion. "Give me your meds and head to bed."

I obeyed.

Early the next morning, I crept out of my bedroom and discovered my sweet sister and Mum, still asleep together. I felt calm, and I began to talk, which woke them up. Immediately, they both started crying and then embraced me, saying, "What have you done? You need help. I have never seen you look this bad."

What I heard validated what I was petrified to hear.

I quickly began to speak and for the first time, I "owned it," that I was sick with an eating disorder, wanted help, and was not at all in control of myself. To my relief, my sister calmly replied, "I know. We know. We are going to get the best help."

I was willing to do whatever to stop this disorder from stealing more of my life and my friends.

Here's some of what I needed to change, and what I realized after the fact. I want to give these to anyone who might identify with even a piece of my story.

****

To consider change, I needed that wake-up call from my friend.

Passing out and being hospitalized were not enough to wake me up; my friend dumping me *with a thoughtful tone* was. Even though I misinterpreted what he said, I knew that he cared enough to tell me something hard. Had he simply disappeared with no explanation, he would have been one of many. My eating disorder made it difficult for me to maintain friendships, to be loved, and to love. I understood this only after I started to heal.

To recover, I needed treatment.

I ended up in a 24/7 setting with others. There, a treatment team helped us to build our healthy selves while disempowering our eating disorders. I was not allowed to use the bathroom for 30 minutes after every meal, and I had all my exercise monitored. My clothing was checked to make sure my disorder hadn't shoved food up my sleeves to avoid the calories. And I had to learn how to talk about hard things. For an entire year I needed THAT level of supervision to break the hold the disorder had on me and let me start finding acceptance within myself.

To be free, I needed to see the lies.

Within eating disorder thinking, almost everything that feels indisputably true is a lie. But while "in it," the lies seemed truer than the truth.

To find me, I had to learn who I was on a much deeper level.

My successes, careers, and diagnoses offered a shell of an identity for a while, and some of it was wrong. For example, I believed I was a "depressed person" because all my life professionals had said it. Instead, I had a full-force eating disorder that caused what looked like clinical depression.

Please be mindful that any labels from others can help/hurt or match/not match. You will find who you are—it can take gentleness and time.

To be whole, I needed love.

I had thought I needed love from certain family members, but I didn't get it as I hoped. I was often the only family-less person at treatment's "family day." I healed anyway. I grew to trust my friends in treatment with me, my team, and my prayers. These eventually lead me to know I was loved, accepted, and worth twice the imaginable.

****

The two biggest benefits of doing the work to recover have been these: first, I no longer feel I need to *prove* myself;

I'm able to *be* myself. Second, I learned how to be loved and give love in a real, wholehearted way.

I married an incredible human being who loves and supports me no matter what. I have a deeply meaningful relationship with my mother, who now lives with us. My sister passed away young, and as complicated as our relationship could be sometimes, I know she loved me, and I loved her. I wish I had realized back then that she always accepted me.

And this leads me to why I stay in recovery even when it's been super hard to do. While in treatment, I met this fantastic light, Georgia. As I was wheeled into the kitchen area on my second day of inpatient, I saw her. She stopped picking off her wild purple nail polish, looked up at me, smiled warmly, and announced, "We're going to be friends." Larger than life, hilarious, real, straightforward, and fabulous, everyone who met Georgia loved her. She became the best friend I had ever had. After I got out of treatment, I'd visit her at different recovery centers. We were not only each other's biggest fans, but friends and chosen family, too.

I lost Georgia to her eating disorder.

Knowing I lost this close, close friend I loved to a disease that I'd felt couldn't touch me? It was a huge awakening. Her death made me fight to keep getting better and staying better.

I'll never know why my precious Georgia lost her battle and I didn't lose mine. Except if I hadn't recovered,

I couldn't love and feel loved like I do. I also wouldn't be so filled with purpose. I still don't totally know *what* my greatest purpose is, but due to my faith, I do the best I can and treat people the way I want to be treated. Right now, that IS my purpose—plus making sure that I offer love and acceptance to my beloved nephew, family, and anyone I interact with.

By the way, I made huge amends with that friend who woke me up back in 2010. I told him how thankful I was for him, and that he made me realize I was not okay when I thought I was. Though his words devastated me then, he saved my life.

Note from Alli:

Our Storyteller, Beau, started off with a weight-loss challenge. As his story stated, he hoped to attain "thin enough" to feel "good enough." Many of us pursue this life-formula, right? However, for Beau, without his knowledge of it, anorexia nervosa unexpectedly took over. When someone doesn't know they have anorexia, they tend to keep pursuing traditional regimens for weight loss such as exercise and dieting/restricting food. These conventional paths towards his goal of weight loss got Beau hospitalized numerous times. He then persisted in searching for what could truly help him to live differently.

We often hear that clinical eating disorders have high mortality rates. This story brings that reality to light. Beau found part of his courage to fight his own disorder because he lost a dear friend to hers.

I felt it was important to share stories that ranged in severity throughout *MeaningFULL*. What each has in common is this: **there is always hope for conquering food, weight, and body image issues, and for changing your problems into life-enhancing perspectives and practices.**

INSIGHTS

IN THIS SECTION, "Insights," the Storytellers offer their hindsight so that it might become your foresight-wisdom. Stories answer, "What I wish I had known about _____ during my food, weight, and body image issues."

I wish I had known about many things, but one stands out above the rest: <u>physiological bingeing</u>. It's the kind that happens when you think you're being weak, but your biology is pushing you to eat. I think if I had known the science behind it, I might have stopped trying to skip meals and limit calories way before I did.

Our diet-focused society rarely highlights this truth, but if you've undereaten, your body will often get you to overeat at some point. Whether that's sooner or later is not in your power. Our bodies are programmed to prevent us from starving, even when our minds want weight loss. If your body is deprived of sufficient fuel to properly and normally function, you can find yourself doing all sorts of food-related things (thinking about food, reading recipes, wanting to touch and talk about food, feeling irritated by others' food related topics, and so on). The underfed body resembles a toddler who's trying to get your attention when you're too busy to give it—persistent and impossible to ignore!

If you feel curious about the various effects of caloric restriction, check out a study that happened more than 70 years ago: the Minnesota Experiment, by Keys and colleagues.[12] In it, healthy males were deprived of calories, probably similar to how many of us diet. The 1948 scholarly journal article, "Observations on Human Behavior in Experimental Semistarvation and Rehabilitation," by Franklin and colleagues[13], offers a succinct report. Although, an old-fashioned Google search may benefit you the most here; it'll likely reveal a plethora of summaries, blogs, and articles pertaining to different aspects of this experiment. Many will be helpful, legitimate, and complimentary (free). To enhance your search results, I've also heard the study referred to as the "Minnesota Semi-Starvation Experiment," "Minnesota Starvation Experiment," and the "Starvation Study."

---

[12] Keys et al., *The Biology of Human Starvation*, (1950).

[13] Franklin et al., *Observations on Human Behavior in Experimental Semistarvation and Rehabilitation*, (1948).

Fitness Through Joy

Billy Blanks Jr.

"YOU HAVE TO be bigger. You gotta be stronger. You have to have a built chest." Males get these messages all the time.

I'm a "skinny" guy, always was, and I love to dance, always have. I've been a professional in the fitness industry since I was a kid. My father, Billy Blanks, created Tae Bo®, and I created Dance It Out®.

In my teen and early-adult years, friends, classmates, adults, whoever (but never my family) would say, "Why are you so skinny?" and "What's wrong with you?" A fellow performer said something I held onto for the first six months of a show: "I don't know why you're so skinny. You look sick." I thought, "Why? Even if I were sick, why would a person say that to someone?" It was just mean.

I wasn't *trying* to be skinny. I was trying to live my life and accomplish whatever tasks I'd set for myself. I didn't understand why people said those things, or what I was supposed to do about them. I got the message, though: I looked weird.

I attempted to fix that once. Trying to gain a little bit of weight, I ate. A lot. I also took protein powder. But my metabolism was just super fast. I quickly realized I was not going to be able to change my basic physique.

I imagine that many reading this can relate to the following: body-shaming remarks, whatever our size or shape, can make us want to cover up. At some points, I hated to look at pictures of myself. I thought I looked too skinny.

In addition to my physique situation, I also got shamed about dancing. In school, I didn't play football. I was the only boy on the dance team, and all the guys made fun of that.

Back then, I tended to interpret some statements literally, and I didn't fully grasp the names they called me. To me, they were descriptions, and the accuracy depended on whether I was or wasn't black, skinny, gay… Hearing those words didn't bother me; the *energy* behind those words did. Just like the skinny-sick comment, I knew what they were saying (or at least how the words felt): "You're dirty," or "You're a horrible person."

Yes, it hurt my feelings sometimes, but I already had an idea inside of me: *it's not my issue—it's theirs.* The shaming stuff they did only made this belief grow stronger and clearer. I'd say to myself, "Wait a minute…" And in that space of reasoning, I'd usually recognize that it was their ignorance or their problem judging me, not something real.

I learned this perspective from my parents, and I teach it to my son. I ask him, "Do they have the power to call you that?" It's like taking a *no* from a person who lacks the authority to give you a *no* about your dream. Once I matured enough to truly realize and practice this, I could tell myself: *"All right, they don't affect me. Just keep going, Billy."* So I did.

I initially started dancing at around eight years old. I would watch Michael Jackson, Paula Abdul, and Janet Jackson on TV, copy all their moves, and show my parents. As I matured, I continued to mimic the professionals' movements. Soon I began performing in live shows. I auditioned for professional jobs right alongside trained, technically perfect dancers. Even when I didn't know what the steps were called, I could do them. (Get this: I ended up playing a ballet dancer in the Broadway musical, *Fame*, discovering the real ballet terms only as I learned them on the job.) Then, one audition changed all that.

I started in the front. The choreographer and dance captain showed us the routine, but I couldn't pick it up fast enough. I went to the second row. Then the third row, the fourth, the back, and then I left. I felt so embarrassed.

My dance-hero stopped me in the hallway. She was so supportive and told me things like, "What's wrong with you? Who cares if these people took classes? It doesn't mean you can't get into classes and grow. You're good, but you're stopping yourself before you've given yourself a chance." She encouraged me to just get *one* of the steps shown, and to do that step with attitude. Gusto. She reassured me, "The other stuff's going to come."

This conversation opened my mind in a whole different way. Repeatedly, I witnessed how dancing scared people. I also knew firsthand that well-trained technical dancers could create an intimidating environment, making you feel like you didn't belong. *How could I help people experience dance as something not scary? Teach that this type of movement is good for you? Show you that you don't have to be a technical dancer to enjoy dance?* Making dance welcoming to anyone, at any skill level, became a mission.

Not too long after I made that commitment, a dance-fitness class I created became the most popular class at the gym. Regularly, 130 came and danced. People told me things like, "Wow! You're changing my life!" and "Your class gives me joy!" Teaching it made me feel happy.

Accomplishing my mission looked promising, but my finances did not. I had a wife and a son, and I couldn't take care of them the way I wanted to. We were homeless and staying in a motel next to the gym's parking garage. I had reached a place where I was ready to give up. Each fitness class paid about $30. I began to think that I was being stupid, that I should go and get a real job-job instead.

The day I went into the gym to tell them, "I'm done," a woman walked up to me and said, "I hope you never stop this class. I cannot explain to you what it means to me." She said all these nice things, then pulled up her sleeve to reveal deep gouges in her arm. She shared that she had a problem with cutting (self-harm), and then she said, "This class makes me not want to do that."

I bawled my eyes out. I realized then, I was not supposed to stop.

And in that moment, in a messed-up way, I felt an inner strength in me, built by the years of shaming comments I had experienced. That familiar reminder came again, but this time from a different, deeply assuring space: *just keep going, Billy.*

Looking back on my journey now, I feel blessed. Several years ago, and with the help of Daymond John and Mark Cuban of *Shark Tank*, I launched Dance It Out (formerly Dance With Me), a dance fitness program that accomplishes my mission. Daily, it allows me to help people find their joy in movement/dance, fitness, and health, which also makes me feel good.

Presently, I'm a fitness consultant to various individuals and on TV. And since I think joy is vital to fitness and overall health, I want to share some thoughts with you here, too.

****

On movement: it's good for you! You have to find your zone.

What is that one thing that you truly enjoy? For some, it may be a sport, like tennis or volleyball. For my dad, it's boxing and karate. For me, it's dance. Moving to music makes me happy, and it makes me feel good. Unless I'm SUPER tired, I never wonder, "Why am I doing this?"

If you don't enjoy what you're doing as "exercise," you'll probably quit it. So find what you like: what makes you feel joy.

On diet: it's about feeling alive.

The word "diet" has such a negative connotation because it's about restrictions. If you make one mistake, you want to jump off a cliff because you think you've ruined it all. I say to "live-it," not "die-it." Choose to eat things that bring life to your body and include pleasure foods. This might look and be defined differently for each of us.

Ultimately, our bodies tell us what's best. For example, I can get super busy, which used to mess up how much and how often I ate. At times, I'd drink five sodas a day and eat nothing but junk (food with little nutrition). Not surprisingly, I'd also experienced headaches, exhaustion, and other stuff. Then about a year ago, I made some food changes in support of my health and some new athletic training I was doing. Forget how I looked; I *felt* different and better than I ever did. So after my training period ended, I kept some of the changes I'd made, just because they made me feel good.

Sometimes focusing on eating for health can get so intense that a person becomes more serious and less joyful. Warning: that's not how it's supposed to go.

On beauty (which includes size and weight): I believe that beauty comes from joy.

Through seeking joy, you find what you love to do. That's going to give you your inner beauty *and* outer beauty; I believe it's the only way that makes a person glow. For instance, I've been around competitive bodybuilders. I was intrigued that, no matter how "perfect" their bodies were, many seemed insecure. I've witnessed that achieving outer "perfection" doesn't promise a glow of confidence or joy; both of those come from the inside.

In my opinion, fitness people should teach about health through the lens of joy. Yes, you want to have a healthy body that you're walking around in. But if you don't have joy, then it doesn't matter. It's like being rich but having no happiness. You might have achieved a perfect body, but if you're unhappy, then what's the point?

****

Thanks for listening to my story and fitness advice. Now that I'm divorced and in my 40s, I've done some living and some lesson learning. I've realized that most of us spend too much time chasing what we think we want, instead of experiencing joyfulness.

I want to spend the rest of my life pursuing what truly brings me joy. This includes the way I feel, the way I look, how I raise my son, how I affect others, and who I am. I wish to feel happy and to appreciate these aspects of me. It doesn't mean that I'm not going to have moments that are not joyful. Even then, at least I can wake up reassured that as a whole, I'm contented with what I'm here to do.

Note from Alli:

Our Storyteller, Billy, started off with body dissatisfaction and body-shame, which he conquered in his unique way: he let it fuel him. As his narrative shows, Billy changed these problems into life-enhancing fitness advice.

I asked Billy to contribute this piece because he and his studio have changed my life. For me, dance meant technique and competition, and fitness meant weight loss and calorie burn. Years of both had burnt me out.

When I arrived at his studio to meet a friend outside, an open house was occurring inside. The music and my curiosity propelled me into the crowded room filled with people sweating and smiling. Two things were immediately clear: fun was happening, and any "diva" attitudes would not be tolerated. (Yessss! Cheering sounds!) For more than an hour, the love of movement I felt from the teachers and students filled me. That was the first time I'd experienced fitness or dance as safe, meaning without judgment from self or others. And years later, the studio continues to bring joy, which keeps me going back for more.

Once, a scale mysteriously appeared in the bathroom. Until then, I had found the space to be one of body acceptance messaging. I left a blunt comment card about it, and poof! The scale disappeared.

The fitness industry can be tricky to navigate since it can include covert and overt diet and weight messages. Practice using your voice; it'll probably become a vital tool in your conquering toolbox and using it can cause positive change.

Lastly and important to your pursuit of overcoming your issues, find exercise you appreciate. These suggestions might assist with how:

- Seek a form of physical activity that evokes an emotional response that's more neutral-to-positive (e.g., "not dread") than negative (e.g., "dread").

- Focus on movement that physically feels (or could feel) enjoyable.

If neither consideration seems helpful and you want movement in your life, try looking for something appealing that connects to an activity. It isn't solely the dancing that keeps me engaged in mine; it's the combination of the camaraderie, creative routines, feeling of safety, sense of accomplishment, and mood uplift I experience each class.

Please be patient with yourself if the approach here seems foreign. Your meaningful exercise could be in the process of unfolding.

My Body Wasn't the Enemy

Anonymous

MY FATHER, AN Orthodox Rabbi and hands-on dad, made sure my siblings and I understood that "God loves you, and there's nothing you can do to change that." My mom had eight children within 12 years and worked full time. With practicality and a smile, she'd explain not getting her nails or hair done: "Your nails and hair are dead."

I grew up in a home with zero focus on dieting, the body, or weight loss. We ate in a balanced way—lots of fresh fruits and vegetables, proteins, starches, and also good amounts of ice cream and treats. So long as it was Kosher, any food was okay.

I was on the slimmer side and an adventurous, healthy eater. I had a good relationship with food. (I would say I had a good relationship with my body, too, but I was still a young girl who wasn't aware of her body yet.)

Like many tweens in middle school, self-consciousness abounded. I looked different because of my hand-me-down clothes. I felt different, too. While most of my classmates lived in multi-million dollar brownstones and penthouses in the city, my family, all ten of us, lived in a basement apartment. I remember I cried on the subway ride home after my 8th-grade pictures. I thought I was ugly with my untrendy, uncontrollably frizzy hairstyle, faded blouse, and glasses.

Right before my freshman year of high school, my mom's friend gave me a compliment that definitely woke me up to the fact that I had a body. We were saying our good-byes while getting ready to move for my father's new job. She announced, "You look great! You've grown taller and lost weight, and you look fantastic. All that baby fat is gone!"

I filled with pride. I stood straighter. I beamed.

Why I was proud baffled me because I hadn't actually done anything to earn such praise. It felt good, though.

A few weeks later, my family settled in, my father met his congregation, and I started my first year at an all-girls, ultra-conservative religious high school. It was much more right-wing than anything I had known. My new and stricter Modesty Code required that long sleeves and tights cover any flesh not concealed by my uniform. No more nail polish or flip-flops. Teachings about God went from loving and positive to "if you don't do this, God's going to punish you."

None of this felt like "me," but I had to do it. For the first time ever, I experienced strife and disconnection with my parents, my culture, and myself. I felt depressed.

That compliment from my mom's friend rang in my ears. Although I wore a junior's size five, I believed that if I could just lose a few more pounds, then that pride, that inner beaming would come again.

I didn't know much about dieting, but I figured it couldn't be that complicated. I understood very little about human physiology, except that the fewer calories I ate, the more weight I would lose. My grand plan was to go on a water diet for a couple of days.

I lasted half a day, and then I broke my water diet. I felt out of control. As soon as I arrived home from school, I raided the refrigerator and kitchen cupboards. I scarfed down food to the point of feeling sick. That was my very first binge.

I had failed at dieting, but I would try the next day again.

And the next.

A dietitian's visit to my 9th-grade class added fuel to my growing fire. Weekly, she taught us how to measure portion sizes and read nutrition labels. When she assigned us to track every calorie for five days, it hooked me! I loved making charts.

After that, I focused on my weight more than the social milestones that my peers enjoyed. I couldn't wait for my driver's license, not so that I could go out with friends to the mall or movies—I couldn't wait to drive myself to Weight Watchers! I spent my savings from babysitting and camp counseling on these meetings, a gym membership, and car insurance. Every day before school, I attended a 5:30 a.m. exercise class.

Still chasing "just a few pounds," I tried every diet plan that existed during the late 1990s and early 2000s. After I got married, I spent even more money on weight loss—which, if I added it all up from youth to adulthood, probably amounted to tens of thousands of dollars. I bought shakes, bars, meal replacements, and packaged foods. I did full programs. One stands out, even today. I ate smoked turkey breast (gross to me) multiple times a day. I powered through it, gagging all the way. I attended fitness camps and boot camps. Most of them happened around the lovely hour of 5 a.m. I trained for a marathon—not for strength or stamina, but in the hopes of losing weight. I hated running.

I worked with professional weight-loss nutritionists. I paid celebrity fees (literally, because I found someone who coached celebrities and sports figures) to have one specific diet coach come to my house each week, weigh me, and give me a meal plan. When the coach arrived, I warned, "This is what's going to happen. I am going to be perfect on the diet, and then I am going to lose control and go crazy. Then I will try over and over again to restart the diet, but I will never be able to get back to it." She reassured me that, "Things would be different this time."

No, things were not. When I broke my diet(s), I went out of control. With a three year old in the car (and you know how hard it is to get in and out with a toddler in a car seat), I would drive myself from one food destination to the next, picking up all my favorite foods—an ice cream store for a milkshake, a bakery for a cake slice with buttercream frosting, a Kosher restaurant with molten cookies and ice cream, another bakery for a croissant, then a coffee shop that had Rice Krispies Treats.

Despite the pain in my stomach that screamed, "Stop eating!" I couldn't stop. I felt crazy! Compelled. Edgy. Angry. How could I be this big of a failure in something so basic? Everybody could successfully diet.

I tried to stop bingeing. In search of support, I shared my experience with a couple of friends, but they didn't "get it." I tried a 12-step support group. The first meeting, I cried with relief because I was finally in the presence of other people who understood. I stayed with this group and my sponsor for a couple of years and even served as the group's secretary, but it didn't help me to stop. I worked with four different generalist therapists for extended periods of time. While therapy was helpful for other things, ultimately, my diet problems and binge eating continued.

Publicly, my husband and I were viewed as a respected couple and loving family in our community. We hosted Shabbat meals. All the while, my pain regarding food was as concealed as my hair, legs, and arms had to be in our culture.

Privately, our marriage suffered from my dieting. Our sex life was in trouble. He was not allowed to touch my stomach or love handles because I felt they were grotesque. Instead of having date nights, I ran off to the support group or weight-loss meetings multiple times a week.

My husband put his foot down. "We are not spending one more penny on diet or weight-loss plans until you go see an eating disorder therapist." I balked at that and told him, "I don't have an eating disorder."

Still desperate to stop bingeing and learn how to stick to a diet, I agreed. I began researching therapists.

Surprisingly, I discovered that nearly any therapist can say they are an eating disorders specialist. However, treating eating disorders is a narrow specialty, and most general therapists are not qualified to do so. With that in mind, I formed questions to evaluate their qualifications. I also checked in with myself as I spoke with each: does this person get me? Do they know what they are talking about?

I interviewed five different specialist therapists. One was not a fit with me, and two seemed inexperienced. I chose the one who felt the most qualified and also offered a brief treatment for 20 sessions called Cognitive Behavioral Therapy for Eating Disorders, "CBT-E." If she didn't work out, I'd go to my second favorite who also seemed to be a genuine specialist, but her approach was long-term.

I began "eating disorder" therapy even though I thought I just sucked at dieting. Almost instantly, I was blown away by what I learned.

****

First, I had binge-eating disorder. I felt mortified and rebuffed the idea. I wasn't really sick like people with anorexia or bulimia. I just had no self-control (or so I thought). I kept imagining that people with real eating disorders would think I was "weak" and didn't belong in the same category as them.

Second, I learned the answer to my questions: "Why couldn't I stick to my diet? Find a diet that worked for me? Lose weight and keep it off?" Because diets don't generally work, that's why! I remember my therapist saying, "80 to 95% of people who go on a diet regain *at least* the weight they lost within five years, others earlier than that." Of course, I spent multiple sessions arguing this from every direction that I could, but she shot back science, which was hard to deny.

I learned that our bodies have a natural set point, a weight that they are happy hanging out at. If we try to go below the natural happy-weight, our bodies rebel and figure out ways to get us back to the weight they want to be.

I learned that restricting food could trigger a physiological binge since bodies tend to fight against the threat of starvation. For example, when I went to London for seminary, I barely ate during the day. Food challenged me there. At night, my roommate and I would devour this African chocolate. I just thought I was weak. No, my body was making up for the calories and fuel I didn't get during the day.

For all those years that I'd thought I had little willpower, my body had just been doing its job. I had lived in a state of guilt for no reason.

Fairly quickly, I had enough science to revise my beliefs. My body was my friend. All those diet "failures" were usually my body trying to keep me healthy and alive. My body wasn't the enemy; the diets were.

****

Gradually, I stopped dieting and bingeing completely. Even so, all those years of unnatural eating caught up with me. I gained about 40 pounds as my body got to its happy-weight.

I won't lie and say that was easy. It wasn't. But I remained committed to the science I had learned. Dieting would only mess up my metabolism even more and make me heavier, which scared me. I had to do my work around my internalized fat-phobia and come face-to-face with my fears about weight gain.

Exposing myself to people with larger bodies helped. Though they seemed atrocious at first, I followed the social media accounts of those who comfortably showed bellies and thighs. Now I see their bodies as just bodies. I've found there's beauty in every body.

I believe that my current weight would be much different had I not ever tried to lose weight. I'm the youngest of three sisters. Each of us started out slim, and I'm the only one who dieted. We recently bought bridesmaid dresses—sizes 0, 2, and I needed a 16. (I *so* wish I could go back to that little 14-year-old me and tell her, "Don't start this, ever.")

I can honestly say that I am happier now—at the heaviest weight of my life—than I was at my thinnest while dieting.

We recently had dear friends visit from out of town. We went to a pizza parlor, which in the past would have been torturous. Instead, it was just my friend and me, ignoring our kids to enjoy each other. When a huge cotton candy arrived at the children's table, I laughed and took pictures. They were giddy with delight, fascinated as the fluffy pink stuff dissolved in their mouths. A few years ago, I would have been focused on the cotton candy and not the kids.

I'm living a full life. Milestones are no longer related to diet or weight. They are beautiful—a loving and respectful marriage, three children whose lives I can be attuned to and fully present for, a great career, and a home where eating is a peaceful time for all of us.

I no longer hide my hair or my body under scarves, sleeves, and tights. The far-right wing of Orthodox Judaism never was me. Instead, I'm negotiating with myself about how I live a religious life. I'm not sure what's going to happen, but I know I'm strong enough to manage. I doubt that I would have gotten to this space of courage without having done the work needed to conquer dieting and discover myself.

If I were able to share only one thing with you from my story, I'd want you to think about this: I wasn't the failure all those years, dieting was. *You are not the failure: dieting is.*

Note from Alli:

Probably like many of us, this Storyteller thought she just "sucked" at dieting and kept trying to do it better. Along the way, binge eating, weight fluctuations, and self-blame crept in, as they often do. Instead of continuing to pursue the ways that were repeatedly failing her, this Storyteller empowered herself. She allowed science to begin to change her mind, which allowed her to eventually overcome her weight-torments, bingeing, and body dissatisfaction issues. The new understandings of her years of distress helped this Storyteller to create a life she valued and preferred.

This narrative introduces a popularly quoted statistic: 80-95% of diets fail. I acknowledge that controversy exists about the exact numbers, but research repeatedly supports that dieting often backfires on the dieter. Many people gain their lost weight within a few years. If you're interested in more information on this topic, the following article is easily accessible online: "Why Do Dieters Regain Weight: Calorie Deprivation Alters Body and Mind, Overwhelming

Willpower," by Dr. Traci Mann[14], a researcher who has studied dieting and health for over 25 years. Also, various listings in this book's Resources section will echo the concept.

The differences between binge-eating disorder and bulimia nervosa can seem confusing since both involve bingeing. During her periods of restriction or exercise compensating for eating/bingeing, this Storyteller may have qualified for another clinical diagnosis: bulimia nervosa or other specified feeding and eating disorders (a catch-all that currently includes atypical bulimia nervosa and atypical anorexia nervosa). The distinctions between each eating disorder can be subtle and sometimes arguable. For more information, please visit the section titled, Concepts and Clarified Terms.

---

[14] Mann, *Why Do Dieters Regain Weight? Calorie Deprivation Alters Body and Mind, Overwhelming Willpower,* (2008).

I Misused These Words and I'm Sorry

Angelica

MY FATHER WAS a cosmetic dermatologist and his brother a plastic surgeon. I spent my teens using a Sharpie pen, circling parts of my body I hated and fantasizing about liposuction.

Born into privilege, my parents insisted on both cotillion and debutante balls. We spent summers at the lake house, held memberships at the country club, the whole deal. Yes, I understand if that makes the following sound whiny: I was so fucking lonely.

I didn't know how to speak about emotions; my culture didn't do feeling-talk. So starting at a very young age, I pieced together an explanation for anything painful in my life: "because I'm fat and ugly." Maybe I did that because my dad pointed out people's flaws as if they had personally offended him with their imperfections, family included. Or maybe it was because I grew up in an uppity area that focused on looks as status. Truthfully, though, I don't know if that culture was any more judgmental than regular ol' society.

Here's what I do know. I misused the words "fat and ugly." Yet as a kid, they were all I knew to say. I have YEARS of journal entries proving this.

I'm a middle of four children and "the sensitive one." My father is volatile, and my mother is submissive. Though present in my family, I was not seen. For example, my mother once found my journal and read about how depressed and "fat and ugly" I was, how I had stopped eating, how I wanted "to die," and that I'd stolen my father's scotch from the liquor cabinet. She punished me for taking the booze and mentioned *nothing* else.

With peers, I was "in" with the popular crowd, and we were mean. (I still feel bad about that.) Throughout elementary school, we ditched friends, cut them off. That is, until one day, they ditched me. No explanation, just the message that they didn't want to be friends anymore. And because of their power in my small private school, this isolated me, which continued for more than a year.

Why did this all happen? I believed, "No one likes or loves me because I'm fat and ugly." Though incompatible with this narrative, I was slightly underweight during those years. That didn't matter.

During junior high, I'd gone from flat-chested and skinny to having hips and big boobs. Suddenly, guys driving past catcalled me. Boys thought they could reach out and touch the big things. I remember this popular kid groping me, aggressively kneading my chest like bread dough. Once he had started, I froze, which apparently signaled to him to continue. He must have interpreted that as me "enjoying it" and bragged to his friends. I hated him touching me where I stuck out, but I felt I had to stay nice to keep him as a friend. I was so alone.

I had already been watching my weight, and that event accelerated it. My teen mind thought: if I can lose the boobs, I'll lose that awful attention. If I can get skinny enough to look or be sick, I'll get attention that feels better. One of my cousins had been through addiction. That taught me that being sick got loving care, even a "deserved" trip to a resort with parents.

In hindsight, I was unequipped to handle sprouting a body that drew sexualized attention. I believed, "People treat me poorly because I'm fat and ugly."

From spring to fall of my blooming-boobs year, I lost an alarming amount of weight and achieved my goal. My mother took me to the doctor who diagnosed me with anorexia nervosa. He didn't recommend that I see a therapist or a dietician or to *talk* about why this might have been happening. Simply, he advised weight restoration as the remedy.

As hoped, Mom doted on me to get well, even brought treats to school to make sure I didn't get hungry. She sweetly requested that I quit my soccer team since the physical activity could interfere with weight gain. I never liked the competitiveness anyway, so I happily agreed. Like my cousin who battled addiction, I got a "deserved" trip, too. I loved these parts of recovery. However, once I had put back on enough weight, the doctor declared me *healed*. Then, my family took on the attitude, "Okay good; she's cured. Let it go."

I had succeeded in fixing one of the two things that were the bane of my problems, and then voila! I was back to "no one cares about me because I'm fat and ugly."

I headed into high school and hoped things would be better. Instead, I got bullied, which included cafeteria foods thrown at me while accompanied by "oink" sound effects. That same year, I also had my first sexual experience, nonconsensual. He had targeted me and made sure I got drunk. I remember people pointing at us and referring to me as the "big jugs girl."

Shortly after that horrible event, we had a holiday brunch, which involved our extended family. I pulled aside my favorite aunt, the one who was always nicest to me, to talk about it. She told me, "Well, you shouldn't have let yourself get drunk in the first place."

I shut my mouth.

I didn't know how to work through the emotional toll of being bullied, raped, and then blamed for being raped. I believed, "It's all my fault because I'm fat and ugly."

I chose a prestigious (of course) college far away from my family, far away from people I knew. Because of experiences up to that point, I'd reasoned: "I'm good only for sex, but at least I'll be wanted." (Makes me squirm now, but that's how my 18-year-old brain worked).

As freshman-year dorm food and chaotic dieting yo-yoed my weight higher, I decided to put my then huge boobs obscenely on display, and a custom pushup did the trick. I would walk around campus wearing ultra-lowcut tops and that bra. I flaunted those things. (The thought of it makes me shiver now—so embarrassing.)

I didn't like the sexualized version of me. Attempting to change it, that summer, I hit Dad up to refer me for a breast reduction, went off birth control pills, and lost weight. Returning to college, I garnered compliments like "You lost weight! You look great."

Finally, I began to feel liked! I began to feel less lonely.

With newfound hope and looking forward to camaraderie, I enrolled in a women's studies course. Being a sensitive person, I tended to tear up easily and cried in class during my presentation on how women's magazines have historically written about feminist movements. When my classmates laughed *at* me, I was stunned and thought, "What the fuck is happening?"

Nothing could save me from the downward spiral—not earning a prized internship at a prominent newspaper, shopping extravagantly, or getting excellent grades. Anorexia took over, and I had to leave school (and give up my beloved internship) to recover. Again.

Once more, "No one likes or loves me because I'm fat and ugly."

After I stabilized and graduated from college, a missed opportunity nagged at me. I hadn't studied abroad like my siblings and peers. I asked if I could spend time in Europe, and my parents agreed to it. They stipulated that I had to work, but they'd pay for me to get there and assist with rent, which was very generous.

Someone I knew lived in Spain, so I decided to go there. She helped me get a job as a barista. As my new employer reviewed my schedule, I blurted out, "When's my lunch?"

I remember that was a turning point for me. With that one simple statement, I'd done two important things: I'd advocated for myself, and I didn't feel guilty for wanting time to eat. Something was already changing inside me on a different level. I would never have done that back in the States.

In Europe, coworkers, customers, and people I met befriended me. They seemed to want my company. It felt easy. They invited me to soccer games and dinners. Women asked me to spend time with them, and they seemed genuinely interested in my thoughts. Some of the married men did hit on me, but I said, "No." More things were changing.

People appeared to like me, and my experiences with them supported that. I could FEEL their regard for me. I wasn't on edge and expecting them to ditch me.

For the first time, I undeniably couldn't match my experience to that usual "because I'm..." narrative.

I recognize that not everyone is going to be able to go abroad to find themselves, and I acknowledge my privilege to do so. Nonetheless, there are some things that, in hindsight, I believe, helped me get free of my food and body battles. I think that any one of them can be considered, started, and done right here at home.

See if you think any might in some way apply to you, too.

****

I needed to feel competent on a level deeper than accomplishments.

I found that making my own money and living independently helped me to feel stronger and more confident.

I needed different experiences.

For example, the culture of truly enjoying food was one I had not tried. There were no calorie lists on menus in Europe, or not that I could read anyway.

I needed to find my community.

I didn't fit the world I was born into. I used to think I needed to change myself (like being mean or ditching people) to feel that I belonged. No, I just needed to find people who liked me.

Since returning from Europe, I found friends here, too. I also found love.

I had tried to push him away by being cagey and noncommittal. But he stayed steady in pursuing me and in treating me with gentleness, patience, and care. My reality no longer matched "nobody loves me." I'm not saying that everybody needs to find a partner or fall in love for everything to go away. But I think that him accepting and loving me helped give me permission to work on being kinder to myself.

Most importantly, I had to fix my language and learn feeling-talk.

I had to stop misusing "fat and ugly" as my own fucked up expressive feeling words. This meant I had to figure out what I was authentically feeling, which was this: loneliness put me deep into a pit of awful, which was dark, toxic, terrifying, and inescapable due to my lack of self-value. That is so different from "fat and ugly."

I had to return "fat" and "ugly" to their dictionary definitions.

This was the easiest one for me.

I choose not to use either nowadays. There are plenty of other words to use. Importantly and to those who strive to stop the demonization of the word fat: I'm sorry for the part I've played in that.

****

Bringing you to today...

After a beautiful stretch with my partner, we have decided to split up. And yes, I'm heartbroken. There's still so much love for each other. Over the years, though, we grew up with, but in different directions from each other.

I'm feeling so lonely because he's been my best and closest friend for more than five years. But the fix for this deep level of pain I'm experiencing is to go through it by talking about it (accurately), crying over it, and experiencing it. I've learned that I'm never actually stuck in that lonely pit of awful; it's just a place that humans visit sometimes.

I've wondered how my life might have been different if I could have talked about my fears and feelings more accurately during my youth. I'll never know.

I'm grateful to not struggle with food or body stuff anymore. Also, accurate feelings and expressions are tolerable. I no longer need to use "because I'm fat and ugly" for everything that goes wrong. That was bullshit all along.

Note from Alli:

This Storyteller, Angelica, repeatedly tried to remedy her life-problems through dieting and changing her body. Though she surgically reduced her breast size and her body frequently changed (even throughout the duration of this short story), neither provided her with lasting, desired results. Her problems eventually lead her to acquire new insight, more precise language, and different ways of being in the world, which helped her to conquer her issues.

This story's repeated use of "fat and ugly" could feel as if I perpetuated the abuse of the words, "fat" and "ugly," which are often used interchangeably and to express feeling states. That was not my intention. To me, this story opens up a necessary discussion that can offer levels of healing and awareness, especially since our Storyteller's thoughts and pursuits are not isolated. All our voices matter. There is value in each of our conquering journeys, including the ones that feel upsetting.

What helped Angelica to overcome her eating and body image issues invites introspection and self-assessment that can serve many people's journeys. If you're open to it, try asking yourself:

- "Do I feel a lack of confidence or competence?" If yes, is there anything, non-body and non-diet related that might help you to feel more confident or competent? Even a smidge of either can do wonders.

- "Am I stuck in my patterns?" If yes, how can you shake up your routines and settings so you can (or have to) pay attention to something new or different?

- "Do I think that no one loves or accepts me?" If yes, I'm betting that someone, somewhere in your life does. It may not be who you want it to be, or like Angelica, you may not know the future. Would you be willing to allow the presence of love or acceptance to help you be kinder to yourself anyway?

- "I am... What?" If your brain tells you that you're this or that, test the accuracy. Here, you might be reasoning something like "I don't choose to think those thoughts; I just kind of hear them. Thus, they MUST be right." Not necessarily! Substituting different vocabulary words for and looking up the definitions of the terms your brain uses can help you test the accuracy.

Any of the above questions might point you in the direction of triumphing over your food and body image stresses. Checking the language that we use to express our feelings and to discuss self (and others, too) can play a vital role in helping any of us bolster our more self-assured, fulfilling lives.

What I Took for Granted

Anonymous

I'M A FREAKING mess. Always have been. I just don't look it. Or, maybe I do. Whatever. Either way, this is me, and here's my story...

From my teens on, I trained as an actress, singer, and dancer. But I didn't strive to become a performer because I thought I was awesome—far from it.

I never fit in socially. In high school, classmates all knew my name because I was absurdly active in clubs, but no one knew me beyond that. Embarrassingly, I didn't understand people my age. Trying to make friends was awkward, confusing, and even debilitating at times. But a pleased director or the sound of an audience clapping? That felt the *opposite*. Pleasing people made me feel liked.

Ever since my first recital, people told me I was gifted at singing, dancing, and acting. In high school, the principal received a letter from a stranger saying I was a "stand out" in the annual musical. I remember deducing, "That letter took effort to write and mail. For a person to go to that trouble, I must have *something* special to offer, even if I have no idea what it is."

Theater seemed the only clear lead for what to do with my life after graduation, and I followed it.

I enjoyed telling stories, especially through music. Hearing an entire auditorium breathing in sync meant we were all on the same ride, as one. Even if it was just for a few hours, *that* intimate level of connection to *that* many people felt incredible.

Selfishly, the stage also gave me a break from my own well-behaved, goody-goody life. I was too immature and innocent to have understood the complex transformation from girl to woman. Once my flat chest grew full and my long, straight legs sprouted curves, I was rarely cast in the "pretty" or "sweet" parts any longer. Instead, I was chosen for comedic, floozy-type roles. I often spoke in a squeaky voice, walked with a wiggle, wore tight clothes, played not bright, or dropped bawdy, double entendre zingers. Truthfully, I didn't know what authentic sensuality was at the time. That being the case, I delighted in making fun of myself as it made others laugh in an "on my team" way. It felt like acceptance, and who doesn't want to be accepted?

Keying into what I thought the media, romantic partners, and my career wanted, my body became an *it.* I believed my worth and work depended on *it,* and I needed to make sure *it* was the best object that *it* could be.

For decades, daily, I devoted hours to the gym and planning what I would and wouldn't eat. Also daily, I spent hours dedicated to my craft: taking classes, doing vocal exercises, memorizing lines, attending coaching sessions, auditioning, keeping up with marketing, and so forth. To stay financially afloat, I waited tables. I set up my life, as best I could, to have every chance of making it in show business.

Fortunately, I worked often as a performer. So much that I remember asking a boss, "Why don't I have any shifts this week?" He said, "Because you keep giving them away." Not shocking, but catering and restaurant managers frowned on me repeatedly getting my schedule covered.

Eventually, more than acting, dancing, or my appearance, I became known for my "high belt," that explosive sound heard in power ballads (and often attempted by intoxicated folks at Karaoke bars). Auditions typically required that I sang songs with those long, loud, emotionally packed notes—all of which, of course, needed to be on key and solid.

No problem! My voice could do it. The rest of the auditioning process was the hard part—hoping the casting people liked me; hoping I was talented enough, funny enough, slim-but-curvy enough, and exactly what they were looking for.

Repeatedly, I made it through multiple "cuts" for my dream parts. (A "cut" is when people either get dismissed or go on to the next round.) After a days- or weeks-long audition process, I'd reach that final-final callback. I'd get nervous. I'd know that only two or three of us remained, that I was probably one round away from landing the role that would validate all the years of hard work. If I got awarded the dream lead or supporting role on Broadway, a national tour, or London's West End, I'd have proof that I'd been something, done something with my life. And, I'd have touched thousands and thousands of lives on the way. Win-win!

The night before, to cope with the wild nervousness, I'd bake something and tell myself, "I'll give it to my roommate," or "I'll just have one:" one brownie, one whatever. Then I'd start eating. The voice in my head would scream, "Stop!" but my hands would keep shoving sweetness in my mouth. I'd eat it all, the whole pan. For a few seconds, I'd feel calmer. Then I'd panic. I had to get back to callback shape. I'd vomit the goods consumed. All of it had to get out of my body.

The next day, I'd wake up, workout, and then do my getting-ready rituals. I'd drink hot liquids, practice scales, and run the assigned songs a few times. My throat would feel tender from hurling, but I never questioned that my singing voice, that belt, would be there, strong and healthy. Why would I? Years of positive feedback about my "powerful instrument" and "huge range" of notes had given me confidence. Plus, my parents and I had spent what seemed like a bazillion dollars on training and coaching throughout the years.

I focused on my appearance because I lacked confidence there.

I'd meticulously rouge, lash, and lipstick myself to suggest the part. Did I look "right" enough? Heels or no heels? Assets highlighted and deficits hidden? One or two pair of tights to suck me in? Did my clothing give a hint of the character but not too much?

So close to fulfilling my dreams. All that work was about to pay off.

I thought that at some point at least the 50/50 would go in my favor, even just statistically. Time and again, I lost those dreamy, life-changing jobs at the end of the audition process. I never knew why.

As I aged, I figured that it was time to finally leave that dream behind and change to another career. I told myself I was ready. I had some great memories. I had done more than most who pursue performing as a career. Though I could share celebrity stories and brag about experiences, I knew my truth: I had failed.

Eventually, I found a career that ignited me. I'd enjoyed my years of food service mostly because of the people I'd met. A few of their stories motivated me to dabble in the world of sales. One thing led to another. Years went by and became decades, but I never lost that nagging feeling of wondering why I'd failed something I'd trained for nearly my entire life.

Around two decades after my last callback, while standing in line at some random bank, I saw the accompanist who played the piano for so many of those auditions. He had become a hugely successful musical director for high-quality and widely visible productions. (Yay him!) My heart raced as I waved to get his attention. He recognized me. We shared rushed pleasantries. At long last, I got to ask: "Why didn't I ever book those parts?" I bit back saying, "Y'know, those life-changing and career-making ones?" He looked at me and said factually, "Your callbacks were inconsistent."

I remember thinking, "Me? Inconsistent? What do you mean inconsi...WAIT."

The light bulb blinked on. Without fail, I'd binged and purged the night before the dream role callbacks. The gymnastics and acid-bath I put my vocal cords through probably made the "inconsistent" part. The more I thought about it, the more obvious the connection. Many of my contemporaries went on to have major theater careers; a few have been nominated for or won Tony awards. I used to make final callbacks with them.

I'm 99% sure the purging destroyed my career. And I have realized something that I want to share with *you*. I wish someone had shared it with me.

****

You may think that there is no consequence of attempting weight control that is unnatural or unkind to your body. And that may be true, but *probably not*. You may be like me and learn about your personal price years after recovery. And my singing career was only one cost.

I rarely say judgmental things like "over/under" and "too much/too little," but I will here. My "overvaluing" of my body's size and shape made me continue "undervaluing" myself. It led me to date people I should not have dated—painful and insulting experiences. It blocked my ability to see that I could have worth in professional, educational, and social settings. And it often made me act out of desperation. I was convinced that I had to work extra-hard to matter. I had to *earn* someone's love by doing things as perfectly as possible and looking the best I could; their praise reassured me I had it. (No one, including me, knew this is what drove my "perfectionism.")

Ironically, I was sometimes sought out and hired for events and even modeling because my "looks" fit a popular mold at the time. This feedback indicated that I had likely achieved that right-enough *it* I had been busting my butt to reach. But I couldn't see it, believe it, or feel it.

I wish I had known that striving to maximize my outside figure could not change any of those internal deficits.

Please don't misunderstand me. I love my life now. I'm fully recovered from yearning to find a body that was as perfect as my limits would let *it* be and from what became bulimia nervosa. Even after the performing completely ended, I couldn't stop my bake-and-barf routine when I felt especially stressed out, and life *is* stressful. (Weird thing is that I had no idea *that's* what I was doing when I was doing it. I still thought my actions were in a justified pursuit of a right-enough body.)

Recovering was not easy, but so worth the work. It gave me the tools for managing life with humor and resilience. I appreciate the earned wisdom that has kept me on the path towards a satisfied life. It's also made my aging process more graceful than it would have been. I find it absurdly funny that an alien appears to have taken over my perimenopausal, hot-flashing body, and has carved lines all over my face.

I no longer rouge, lash, and lipstick myself. I feel prettiest and most "me" with little to no face painting.

Compliments and positive feedback (I no longer hear clapping) now feel like what they are, nothing more.

I recognize that emotions are what they are. I'm still alive and able to smile after having experienced many grotesque feelings now.

I'm still "a perfectionist" because I like pushing myself. I now have a choice about when and what. For instance, I choose messy cupboards and computer desktops.

It took a while to stop looking at my body as an *it* instead of *me; we are one.* Nowadays, I'm grateful for health.

****

I don't regret anything at this point because everything in the past is an ingredient of life in the present. Having said and meant that, I confess: I occasionally find myself wondering how far I could have gone in the stage world if I hadn't boxed myself in like I did. I was willing to pay nearly any price to try to reach that good body, that object. And frankly, that made me less confident, less talented, and less happy.

I wish someone had told me this story a long time ago. So I'll ask you now: do you have a belief that the rest of your life depends on? If so, please question it. Make sure yours isn't something cock-eyed that your younger mind put together as best it could.

Note from Alli:

This Storyteller tried to manipulate her body into fitting ideas about what she, others, and possibly an industry determined was "right." Traditionally, dieting and exercise would be sound ways to reach her goal of a "right" body, and she did those with vigilance. She added purging too. Eventually, she realized that what she believed would help her wasn't doing that. She then worked to recover from the beliefs and behaviors that diminished the quality of her life and had become bulimia nervosa. By figuring out who she was inside, by adding more flexibility to her perfectionism, and by gaining wisdom about her life-formulas, she gradually unlocked a fuller existence.

Instead of the more common physical consequences that can come from purging, this Storyteller encountered unexpected damage from it: her career. This reminds us that we're each unique in how we experience the consequences of our struggles (and our triumphs, too!).

This story also introduces the pressure that can come from being in certain environments. People are going to participate in different looks-and-physique-focused industries (e.g., certain athletics, beauty pageantry, acting, and modeling). And people are going to be exposed to areas in life that are rife with pressuring messages (e.g., social media, the magazine end cap at the grocery store, various health care settings, and sometimes our homes). I invite you to consider the following:

- Which of your environments most affect your relationship with food, weight, or body image, and how so?

- Could you alter or challenge your setting to better support you? For example, on social media, maybe limit your time or don't visit sites that trigger self-hate. In a health care setting, try asking your provider for recommendations that have nothing to do with size or weight.

For this Storyteller, she possibly could have challenged her environment's influence on her by choosing to pursue a role that didn't focus on her body. Sometimes simply mixing up the status quo can help you to find a new perspective within you.

Each of our solutions and salvations will be unique. But awareness about what amplifies our dieting, weight, and body image issues can serve us, helping us to find more relief from our food and body pressures.

Unexpected Obstacles

Staci Lawrence

A LIFE INSURANCE underwriter denied me their highest level of protection—because of my BMI.

I am a nonsmoker who's physically active and eats the "rainbow," as the posters in the doctors' offices say. My mom died young from a genetic disease, and that did count against me too. But, really, my weight mattered as *the* thing. The underwriter said the decision-makers wanted me to gain 30 to 40 pounds to be "healthy" enough to be insured.

I'm skinny—always have been.

In middle school, kids would chase me down in the snow, circling me, threatening and pushing me. I looked like I couldn't protect myself. It wasn't that I *couldn't* protect myself; I *wouldn't*. I was that kid who got regularly picked on because I wouldn't fight or be mean back. Those kids taught me I was not just "skinny" but a "skinny *bitch*."

I'm now in my 40s. It's so interesting how "skinny bitch" has continued throughout the years—just with a different tone.

Like a lot of moms, I wake up, wake the kids up, and dress myself in wrinkled gym-clothes grabbed from the dryer. I don't want to work out, but I have to. I kiss my second child good-bye at school, I speed to the gym to cram it in before work. I want to be strong. I want to know that in an emergency, I can scoop up my children and run. My mother died from high blood pressure in her lungs. She became unable to catch a breath, and that scares me for my future. So, working out is important to me.

Every time I mention to a certain friend that I'm headed to the gym to meet my trainer, I hear, "Oh, you bitch, I don't know why you're wasting your money on that. You're so lucky, YOU can eat." I'm used to it now. I wait for the subject to change. I don't say anything snarky because I try not to ever actually *be* a bitch (unless it's necessary, that is).

I have not spoken about my experience or my body-privilege before right now. I know people can feel annoyed by very thin people, and I might be perceived as whiny or ungrateful—even worse, my experience might feel hurtful to someone. Yet, I'm not alone in the following: living outside the BMI's "normal" range comes with unexpected obstacles.

Being skinny influenced my job pursuits in ways that required adjustments.

Once I moved to Hollywood and began auditioning for television shows, commercials, and movies, my acting skills were validated, so my training and talent fit in. But what was the *rest* of the feedback?

"She didn't seem like she had the body to be a mom, but there's this drug addict role..."

"She doesn't look like she could be a Midwestern Mom with two kids." (Seriously? I **AM** a Midwestern Mom with two kids!)

I have now proudly played: a degenerate, an addicted mom, a person recovering from anorexia, and a meth dealer. (In Hollywood, work is work and I'm grateful for it. At least they're interesting roles!)

My thinness derails medical attention.

Before they meet me for the first time, medical doctors see my height and weight. Without fail, they come in with, "Soooooo [exhales], is this a normal weight for you?" I, smiling, reassure them, "This has been my weight since high school."

I know these discussions are coming from a place of care, but it sends me into a tailspin of, "I left the house feeling normal. The doctor seems concerned. Do I look that weird?" Frankly, I don't want to waste time on if I'm eating enough. I want to get to the real reason I'm there: help. I made the appointment for something unrelated to my weight.

My thinness counted against me when applying for life insurance.

As mentioned, I was supposed to gain 30 to 40 pounds to be awarded the highest level of protection for my family. But no matter what has gone on in my eating and exercise, I have never been able to significantly change my body weight. I've tried! Here's the most extreme example, which was not while I was actively attempting to gain weight. On stage during a play, I had to eat 13 pieces of pizza every night for two weeks. I ate how I usually ate during the day before the show. I did not gain anything but water-bloat.

This might sound dreamy to some, but not to me. Gaining even two pounds (which I proudly and recently did), I have had to dedicate *so much* mental and physical energy to it—like hours and hours a week. To what extremes and how UNhealthy would I get while trying to add 30 pounds to my frame?

I felt outraged that I couldn't take care of my family because my body wasn't in the "normal" weight range of some chart. My mind raced with all the times I'd heard, "You're one of my healthiest patients." And since there was no way I could meet the underwriter's expectations, I set out to prove that I was "healthy" by getting those same doctors to write letters on my behalf.

After a preposterous amount of effort, I finally got the life insurance I had applied for. And here, I really see the privilege of thinness. I've heard that people outside of and on the other side of the BMI may not be able to get the doctors on their sides like I did. And I think that stinks.

My thinness created a lifelong sense of not-enoughness.

People I barely know say, "Oh you're so skinny!"— like it's a compliment. But it's not; it usually comes with what feels like resentment. When it comes from a friend, I want to apologize for my body. And when it comes from a stranger? I want to say something super fucked up (or inject some awkward dark humor) to teach a lesson: "That's the problem with chemo," or "Yeah, I haven't eaten in 7 months; makes me cranky." No, I would never do that, but I *want* to.

After a lifetime of these kinds of obstacles and messages, I think anyone would start trying to make sense of it. *So I am too skinny to be attractive. I'm a goofy, thin chick. I look ill. I'm a skinny bitch. I'm weak and fragile.* At different times, each got inside me. I fought to not believe them as best I could.

It's taken years to fix those insecurities. I remember reading an article about a parent who unwittingly gave her body-insecurities to her child. That woke me up. Realizing I'm my daughters' female role model, my mission has become showing love to others and loving myself. I had to put my insecurities on display (not easy) and work through what I could—towards self-love. Change has not been simple or immediate. But here's how I think I did it (and am still trying to do it, daily.)

****

I aged, which has done so much for me.

There's an inherent growth that happens. With every decade, more self-assurance seems to come.

I accepted the discomfort of being in this body.

People are going to say things about it. I remind myself that those comments are not about me, they are about their pain—their having been attacked simply by living in their body, their oppression, whatever things they are going through.

I recognized that if I'm choosing to live a "healthy" lifestyle, then I'm choosing to do things that make me feel empowered.

I'm on a never-ending quest for more flexibility—both figurative and literal. I've been working on both my body's and mind's limberness for years. I tune in to how foods and drinks affect me—I haven't had soda since I realized it gives me a headache between my eyes. I work out because it makes me stronger. I try to live each day with a sense of purpose, positive relationships, joy, and being in the present moment.

I faked affirmations, trying to believe them, which I eventually did.

I had to convince myself: *I'm beautiful. I'm enough. I love my body. I love my face. I love my life.* It's that idea that you tell the universe what you want, and the world will conspire to give it to you. And I, like probably anyone else, also needed someone to reflect self-love at me. For me, it's a good therapist and my friends; for others, it might be a pastor, mentor, or a partner.

I worked through some of my painful and uncomfortable stuff by doing stand up comedy.

I once went to the doctor about a scary lump in my breast. After examining me, she deadpanned with the finesse of a pro, "You actually have to have breast tissue to have breast cancer." The lump? It was my rib. Yep, that made it into my act.

My biggest change came from becoming a mother.

I looked at my children and saw perfection reflected back at me. I realized, "How can I think I'm anything 'less than' when these children are so precious?" They are made with my husband's genetics and mine. Both kids have my smile that I regarded as "gummy." Their smiles are not gummy; their smiles are beautiful. One daughter has my forehead. I always thought mine was too big for my face. Her forehead is not too big for her face; hers is perfect. The other has my narrow palate and crooked teeth. They both look like me; they both look like him. Through our eyes, they are perfect, pure, and beautiful young people.

****

Seeing my children and life through a mother's eyes, *that* has made me feel more whole and (I never thought I'd say and mean this) beautiful, myself.

185

Because of what I have been through, I am vigilant about honoring all bodies and teaching my children to respect all bodies too. I can't do much to change what happens outside my house, but I can teach my kids not to perpetuate appearance biases and body comments. My husband and I do not talk in a way that places value on body sizes. We teach our daughters: *you don't comment on things that people don't choose. Like if you see someone with acne on their face, you say nothing. But if you notice a friend who changed their hair from natural to pink, and you think it's totally cool, then go for it. Share how awesome you think their self-expression is.* I hope that these lessons might help them to grow up well and also to improve things for anyone they meet whose body, face, shape, or whatever is different than "normal."

Thank you for allowing me to have a voice about my experience. I'm sure I'm not alone.

Note from Alli:

Our Storyteller, Staci, struggled with the problems of being not at a "normal" weight and experiencing body shaming because of it. Instead of trying to change her body in ways that would likely be unsustainable, Staci discovered personal realizations that enabled her to overcome her issues and to enhance her interactions (especially with her children). Staci still receives body-shaming messages.

I feel embarrassed to share this, but I first felt surprised to learn that Staci's thinness triggered some similar-ish hurdles that a person in a larger body can experience (e.g., original denial of life insurance level and people assuming negative traits about her because of her weight). Admittedly, thin privilege affects her experience. That said, when I was testing out the narratives with readers, I noticed this story elicited reactions ranging from feelings of annoyance and jealousy to gratitude for including skinny-shaming in this collection. If you had emotional responses, please don't judge yourself (or our Storyteller). Just notice.

Numerous scientific articles have pointed out that the BMI chart does not indicate health statuses with accuracy. If you'd like to review a summary of the problems with relying on the BMI (e.g., outdated, does not account for bone size or muscle mass), check out the National Public Radio's 4-minute listen, "Top Ten Reasons Why the BMI is Bogus," by Keith Devlin.[15]

I ask you: if an elite athlete who is at their peak can end up in the obese or overweight categories according to the BMI, is it possible it could be wrong about you, too?

Lastly, even if you have seemingly no breast tissue like this Storyteller, her checkup results may not be yours. Anyone can get breast cancer—males, too. Although Staci's medical doctor joked with her about her situation, you still need to get any lumps in your chest area examined.

---

[15] Devlin, *Top 10 Reasons Why the BMI is Bogus*, (2009).

Live Fully

Laura James

I COME FROM sturdy stock, hitting 350 pounds at my biggest. After bariatric surgery 15 years ago, I stayed hovering around 250 pounds even with an active lifestyle. I say these numbers because I want you to know that I am a person who lives in a larger body. This story, however, is not for exclusively larger-bodied people. This is for *anyone* whose body image or size holds them back from living how they want to.

STIGMA EXPERIENCED

Sure, I've been made fun of because of my body. When I was young, the eye rolls and weight comments would get to me. I mean, puberty isn't fun for most anyone, but even more so for a young girl already in "plus-size." I had convinced myself I was an introvert (preferred being alone). Really, I was avoiding the pain of being picked on. Kids could be horrible!

As I grew older, the teasing decreased (thank god people mature), and I formed a sense of resiliency to it. Any time I'd hear a "moo" sound or a cow comment, my eyes would roll exaggeratedly. I'd wonder, "What motivates a person to do something like that?"

They were definitely the weirdos, not me.

FEAR OF JUDGMENT

So, there I was, mostly steady in believing that if someone does something rude or cruel (not to be too cliché), that says more about that person than it does about me. After all, this is the only body I get. Attacking it/me for simply *existing* in the world???

Yet I'd sometimes still feel trapped by fear. Who was going to judge me? Point at me? Pick on me? Reject me? I'd make decisions based on my size and how I felt about it—parties I didn't go to, clothes I didn't wear, and chances I didn't take.

I know that I'm not alone in this. And I know people of any weight go through similar insecurities. We're human, and let's face it; putting ourselves out there feels scary sometimes.

ACTUAL LIMITATIONS

I vividly remember myself leaving a well-known plus-size retail store in tears. I could not find a single pair of pants—in the whole store—that would zip comfortably, and I needed appropriate slacks to attend a work event. In the dressing room, I started crying, panicking. "What do I do next? I now don't deserve clothes that fit me because of living in *this* body. I can't go to the event because of living in *this* body." I felt humiliated.

I'd spent my whole life on and off diets. My mother, father, and brother were all "heavier," too, so whatever was trendy, whatever the women's magazines had posted, we did—and of course, Weight Watchers. Once I left home, I continued efforts to reduce my size.

I know this may sound difficult to believe, but when I relaxed and didn't diet, I didn't eat *a ton*. I didn't ever "binge" or have an eating disorder. I would, however, sometimes eat for comfort, and as a professional chef, I appreciated rich foods. I ate similarly to the medium and small-bodied people who surrounded me, with the difference being their "medium" versus my "large" order. I had an active job (think of any of those popular chef-competition TV shows), and I also worked out, taking step aerobics classes at least three days a week. Had I been a small-bodied person, people would have probably described me as having "an appetite" but "living an active lifestyle." However, I wasn't a small person. I was stuck in my body, trying to live a "normal" life while not being "normal"-sized.

At that moment in that dressing room, I realized I was either going to the work event inappropriately dressed, naked, or not at all. HOW could a plus-size store have *nothing* for my body? After enough tears and berating myself, I wore overly casual pants from my closet to that "dressy business" event.

THE SOLUTION (NOT SO MUCH)

At a later point, a bunch of celebs on TV had introduced the new weight loss rage—bariatric surgery. In front of my eyes, they shrunk. I had found my solution, or so I thought. Desperate to live easier, do all my activities more easily, and to get to a more "normal" body, I decided I'd have a Roux-en-Y surgery: I'd have a piece of my stomach cut out. Afterwards and as predicted, life did get easier while a bit smaller. I felt so excited the first time I could cross my legs. Although it was lovely to fit in chairs with armrests, to move unobstructed through narrow aisles, and to jump higher in my fitness classes, my surgery had a short-lived benefit and a lasting cost.

One of the side effects for me was poor vitamin absorption. I now deal with anemia, which knocks down my energy level. I also have to undergo occasional iron infusions and regularly monitor my levels. On top of all that, the surgery was never as "successful" as was promised. I regained most of the weight.

What. The. Hell.

So yes. I've had my share of struggles and have empathy for any size-related struggles you go through. I get it. And on the other hand, I have also grown stronger and stronger about not letting my size hold me back.

LIVING FULLY

I face myself daily, and so I feel thankful for a unique upbringing that allows me to live in the following truth: I will not wait for my body to be smaller to do things and live fully. Otherwise I will miss out on life.

My whole family, especially my father, strongly valued "living fully." Dad always role-modeled "normal" living no matter what our sizes. He was ever-present on the basketball court and in the pool. His gym bag was always in the laundry room, ready to be washed for the next day's game or swim. Early on, he pushed me to start sports. I discovered that I loved to swim, and even became an instructor. I played a lot of basketball and softball, too. I simply loved being athletic: the way it felt to move, to focus on a ball or on beating a time, and to push my body to its max. I wasn't ever the star player, but I was a team player for sure.

Since discovering this part of me, I've never shied away from physical activity, even when weight stigma could be present; the benefit makes me encounter any potential risk head-on. I remember taking a paddleboard lesson with my good friend and activity-buddy. To stand up on the board, I'd have to kneel first, then bring my feet under me to "pop" up. While I think I'm pretty flexible, *that* combination was not happening. I couldn't get my limbs to move fast enough. Each time, I'd fall off. Then the instructor would help me back onto the board. He'd suggest a different way we might get me up. Each time, I'd get close, then splash!

Though it was frustrating not to nail it, we had a great time and laughed a lot. I also felt no judgment from the instructor. No, "Oh, I'm having to help this fat chick" attitude. Instead, he genuinely seemed to support my determination.

You might think I sound "brave." Maybe you think I'm Pollyanna. Maybe you are calling "bull" right now. I get these reactions about my attitude, and that's fine, because here's the deal. I'm clear about what I want in life: experiences and fun memories.

I recently turned 50, and the benefit of age and hindsight has brought a lot of insight.

****

I've learned that I gain nothing from avoiding things I want to do, and I can gain A LOT from trying new things.

Though I was totally against it, Dad pushed me to join a sorority. I had predicted that the girls would be bitchy to this introvert. To the contrary, I discovered the sorority sisters were great, and social life suited me—too much! I didn't graduate from college. I was too busy *not* going to class to instead be with sisters and friends. Plus, I figured out there were boys who don't care about what size a girl is. Of course, I enjoyed that, too. I'm glad I didn't hold myself back from sorority life because, through it, I discovered the "real me" is an extrovert.

I've learned that I value experiences more than I care about potentially being judged.

That same activity buddy invited me to her boot camp class—lots of weightlifting and running around. While doing each station's tasks (burpees, jump lunges, squats), sweating buckets, and enjoying myself, I overheard my friend telling the instructor, "She is ready to try anything." I paused to think about it and realized for the first time: I *am* ready to try anything, whether pre-bariatric, post-bariatric, this weight, or that weight. It's an attitude that has given me lots of pleasant memories.

Another example: I've recently begun performing on stage in musical revues. Under the direction of a professional, a bunch of adults with all sorts of careers and backgrounds "put on a show" and invite an audience. What a rush to dress up in a costume and perform on a real stage! For a girl whose only prior theatrical experience had been a rifle-twirling drill team stint back in high school, how else—but by being willing to try anything—could I have had this kind of opportunity?

I've learned that people will say things about me and my body. (Although they're not always negative or what I expect.)

Both behind my back and to my face, I've heard people call me "inspirational" and "fearless" because I'm always out there doing things and enjoying life. To be honest, I bristle a little at either. Both set an expectation that anyone with a body that is not "average" is inspirational for just going about their life. On the other hand, I feel glad that I can encourage people to not stop themselves from doing what they want to do.

I've learned that if I make an effort at something, it will reward me in some way.

Heck, after auditioning for my fourth performance series, the vocal director deemed me "most improved" at singing, which made me feel like I could accomplish *anything.* Singing on key was a HUGE challenge for me (and had absolutely nothing to do with my size).

Listen, I have insecurities and indecision like anyone. But I also know I can work through both, by talking through them with friends. And I'm glad I do that, because the experiences and memories have been worth it.

At my highest-highest weight, I met my husband (love him), made a successful career change, and extensively traveled for work. Through having to get from point A to point B alone and often, I think I built a ton of self-determination. If I needed a seatbelt extender, I either brought one myself or unapologetically asked for one. What else was I gonna do—not fulfill my job's assignment? So it kind of made me get over apologizing for having needs.

****

Because I've been through a lot with my own body's stubbornness about size, I tend to notice other people's pain out there, and there's a lot of it. I see how upset people get in the dressing room area because nothing fits or fits right. Instead of berating yourself for it, maybe start questioning why there aren't more size and style options available for **all** of our diverse body sizes and shapes.

Hopefully some of these thoughts can help encourage and support you. Be safe about it but honor *you* and the life you want. Stop waiting for your body to change; get out there and live fully.

Note from Alli:

This narrative applies to anyone who feels shame about their body not being what they want it to be. I believe we conquer this more by getting out there and "living" than trying to morph our physiques into unsustainable forms. Our Storyteller, Laura, could have let her body and people's shaming hold her back from living a life she loves—many (of any size) would do so to avoid potential ridicule. Instead, Laura overcame her problems by learning about herself and putting those lessons into action.

Granted, Laura's life force and enthusiasm are unique. I met her during the musical revue she mentioned, and I've personally witnessed people's biases and discrimination in action, directed at her. I've watched her refuse to let that deter her from experiencing each moment.

She inspired me to think about how she does this. She seems to have a capacity for tolerating and accepting feelings, both hers and others, without judgment. Add these skills to her appetite for experience and her clarity of intention, and she's empowered.

Please don't compare yourself to her. As stated, Laura is a one-of-a-kind (as are you). Additionally, if you find yourself wanting some of that resilience mentioned—some of that "You can think what you want, and I'm here to do what I'm here to do" attitude—here's an exercise for you.

- First, accept your own feelings, right here and now, about this story. If you feel in disbelief, if you feel annoyed, if you feel defeated, if you feel inspired, if you feel hopeless, if you feel skeptical—let those feelings be with you, without judging them.

- Next, think about whether there's anything in this piece that connects with you. Maybe you want more courage, less fear of judgment, or more clarity about your own goals and intentions.

- Now, imagine yourself on that paddleboard and wearing your bathing suit. Imagine the eyes on you while also staying focused on figuring out how you'll "pop" up to stand. Allow your brain's chatter to exist. Same with the feelings that come for you. Don't judge either, and get yourself to try to stand up on that board.

Even in imagination, you may not feel confident YET. Practice accepting your feelings (so you can know yourself), letting what's deeply important to you influence your decisions, and focusing on your intentions for what you want to create in your life. These tools can help you to conquer your eating and body image issues.

MEANINGFULL

This is one of the rare stories that mentions numbers. In this case, Laura and I decided that they could exist for clarification.

CONNECTIONS

IN THIS SECTION, "Connections," stories from family, friends, and teachers answer, "How _____ is different now that someone I care about seems free or freer from their food, weight, and body image issues."

Because preoccupations with dieting, weight, and body are seen as so normal in our society, it can feel like no one notices what you're going through when you're going through it. This section reminds us that people who care often do see you, including your pain and joys. They may be there for you and with you right now.

A Matter of Life and Death

JD Ouellette

I RAISED MY kids alongside a sea of tan, lithe women in tennis clothes moaning, "I hate my thighs." For decades, I puttered along, tinkering with food intake, weight-loss meetings, and diet foods, feeling noble and purposeful when I stuck to diet and exercise routines. And then, my normal life entered a terrifying twilight zone.

Virtually overnight, our outgoing, bubbly high-school senior moved from a carefree, energetic, take-the-world-by-storm teenager to someone who moved robotically through her days. While watching my child inexplicably fade before my eyes, I knew something was horribly wrong.

Keep in mind, I had my own background leading up to this (as most of us probably do). I didn't originally react when she began a "healthy eating makeover." Who would? It sounded so positive and was not focused on her weight but her health.

I had been the thin child of a svelte, gorgeous mother who was single and on welfare with two babies in 1966. To understand the culture of the time, think of any television series set in the '60s and '70s where stunning secretaries understand the following: open judgment of their bodies by boorish bosses is the unwritten part of their job description. To fight for a better economic life, my mother fretted over her aesthetics. She forbade sugar in our home and lived off an instant breakfast drink, coffee, and cigarettes during the day. She ate only at night and would check her belly size by touching it. She'd say she was "bad" if she ate with enjoyment.

As I moved up the numbers at the size 5-7-9 clothing shop and into the body of a curvaceous young adult, my mother would oh-so-lovingly remind me, "You want to be sure you never hit size 11." However, I was meant to have a generous body, one that was on the sturdy side just like my mother's mother.

In my twenties, the doctor said, "Wow! You'd never know by looking at you that you weigh this much. For your height you should be 20 pounds lighter." I remember thinking, "That's a weird thing to say" because I felt healthy and all my laboratory tests fell within the normal range. Regardless, my weight didn't match the "ideal body weight for height" number on a chart.

Between the medical professional's judgment and my family culture's rule of "fear and fight fat," I decided to do what one is supposed to do when one's body doesn't conform to the ideal. Over the following years—marked with dating, marriage, and children (two boys and two girls)—I settled into a lifestyle of restricted food intake, of cardio on the elliptical and a varying circuit of weight machines, and of trying to convince myself that I liked no-fat foods.

As a "stay at home" mom and "professional volunteer," I had the life I wanted, just not that "ideal" body to match it. I would never call what I did in pursuit of thinness "enjoyable." Regular exercise was a chore in service of weight loss. The result? My weight most successfully yo-yoed.

Unlike my own childhood, I mindfully tried to keep diet-talk and weight messages out of our home. I absolutely did not speak about my own dieting or relationship with my body. My husband and I taught our children to think critically about messages the media communicated. We listened to their music and watched their TV with them, discussing themes that objectified women.

At every weight (and there were many), I hiked, kayaked, and swam with my family. I did this both to set a good example and to join in the fun. All the while though, I silently fretted and felt self-conscious about my body.

In American culture, the body represents status, and the thin ideal appears the ultimate in both health and aesthetics. And although I never said it out loud, this educated, proud feminist could not stop feeling *lesser than* because I didn't have the "right" body. So I subtly kept watching what I ate and exercising to get mine closer. All that changed when I noticed my daughter beginning to change.

At first it was small things. She suddenly had no interest in Winter Formal or doing things "one last time" with lifelong friends. "Social Butterfly," a nickname she had rightfully earned, stayed home on weekend nights instead of at football games or senior-year parties. When I first asked why, she made excuses; she wanted to spend more time with me and her father before leaving for college, and there was "too much partying" senior year. On the one hand, we congratulated ourselves on raising such a sensible, loving girl. On the other, we knew this was out of character and odd.

Things got weirder and scarier. She told me a hard-boiled egg was a "full meal" and inexplicably needed to cut it into 64 small cubes to eat it. My suggestion that an egg wasn't enough to constitute a meal resulted in a screaming match over autonomy.

As baffling as that was, when her doctor expressed concern over her sudden weight loss and changed vital signs (likely from her inefficient nutrition), her nonplussed attitude was surreal. It is almost impossible to explain the terror that began to grip my heart and soul, hearing her argue that nothing was wrong with her. She was simply doing a "healthy eating makeover." She justified her target weight as "realistic" because she had friends that weighed that. (Yes, but they were eight to ten inches shorter than she was!)

Her flat demeanor in the face of our rising anxiety made everything familiar about her and our relationship unfamiliar overnight. On a college visit, she declared that there was nothing in the gourmet salad and pizza place she could possibly ever be expected to eat and stormed out of a restaurant. She left her father and me with our mouths agape—and with tears in our eyes. Navigating daily life with her felt like someone had rearranged all the furniture in our house, in the middle of the night, and cut the power on top of that—nothing was familiar.

Four terrifying months stretched between the beginning of a diet to the beginning of her treatment and recovery. Doctor's visits, medications for stomach pain, and bizarre interpersonal conflicts filled the interim. Manipulations and red herrings from her abounded. (It's part of how the illness affects someone.) My wanting her to eat more than a handful of blueberries became accusations of "you're just afraid of an empty nest." Everything was "your problem," (i.e. *my* problem) and not hers. We all shed tears during this time.

Eventually, frantic Googling about anorexia nervosa provided an avenue to explore and a seemingly valid explanation. Fortunately, our pediatrician was up-to-date and knew where to refer us—even advocated for coverage with our insurer.

With laser focus, I listened to our treatment team at the University of California San Diego. My daughter was diagnosed with anorexia nervosa, explained as a largely genetic and neurobiological disorder involving a malfunction with the brain's reward center pertaining to eating and anxiety. Her "healthy eating makeover" had put her in a state of negative energy balance (a status where energy output is greater than energy/calorie intake). UC San Diego would use a treatment model called FBT or family-based treatment. In this approach, "food is medicine," and my daughter was going to need thousands of calories of medicine per day for her specific treatment plan. She would require lots of fat to heal her brain, which had been deprived of enough fuel and nutrients. Deep down, and now recognizing the terror anorexia nervosa engenders in its targets, I knew that she would need her mother to help her eat and gain weight.

Love led me to cultural disobedience. Concern around my own weight control went out the window—along with low-fat anything. Maximum fat and calories were now the weapons with which I would fight for my daughter's life.

Our first meal, a real one with pasta and cheese and bread (not the abomination of a single boiled chicken breast she had been calling dinner), I stood up to her anorexia. I spoke directly and firmly to my daughter locked inside the disorder, "If I have to gain 50 pounds for every five you gain, I will do it in a heartbeat." And I meant it.

Her diagnosis flipped a switch in me. Although anorexia and dieting are completely different (one might be conceptualized a metabo-psychiatric illness and the other is viewed as a culturally-normed "healthful" practice) they both share a behavior: food restriction. Eating with a concern for my own weight could no longer be a part of my life AT ALL; *her* life depended on that.

As a side effect of her anorexia nervosa, which took three agonizing years to fully remit, I went on my own dieting-recovery journey. Unexpectedly, helping her to heal repaired my own childhood issues with my food and body.

Today, I am a 55-year-old professional woman, wife, mother, grandmother, an eating disorders and social justice advocate, and at peace with myself, including with my body. My weight has been seven-years steady at "IDGAF" (I Don't Give a—insert the "F" word here that works for you).

****

My diet and health epiphanies were these:

- Through learning about the Health At Every Size® movement, I realized the endless holes in both the science behind and conventional wisdom around weight and health. Who knew that "overweight" people have been shown (in scientific, peer-reviewed research) to live longer than any other weight category?[16]

- I discovered that my weight is no proxy to measure health. Instead, mood, energy, and various lab tests tell me things no scale ever could.

---

[16] See **Note from Alli** for this journal article reference.

- I moved past a lifetime of disordered messages. I reached a conclusion that appearance-based healthcare is not healthy for my family and me.

- I discerned physical and mental health as equally important. Overvaluing one shortchanges the other and knocks wellness out of equilibrium.

- After reflecting on the baffling custom of having scales in homes and using their numbers to serve as guides for how we are to view ourselves, I was able to view it as arbitrary and ludicrous. Obviously, my worth is not my weight!

- I rediscovered the shocking truth that when I approach food with no restrictions in mind, no calorie counting, and no moral judgments around food choices, I spend a fraction of the time thinking about food! It is a freedom I had not had since I was a skinny teenage field hockey player, scarfing cheese fries with friends after a game.

My exercise epiphany was this:

- When I measure a successful workout regimen by how I *feel* versus what I hope to accomplish in terms of weight loss, exercise is not a chore but an important part of maintaining all-around health.

My cultural epiphany?

- "IDGAF" about how my size or shape fits in American culture!

Needing to heal from the stress of my child's life-threatening illness, I integrated all I had learned and moved forward in an improved normal. Each of these epiphanies has made life better, fuller, and freer.

****

My daughter is now seven years out from beginning treatment. This happy, healthy, young woman with two college degrees is fulfilling her childhood dream of working in law enforcement. She is halfway through our regional academy, on her way to becoming a Deputy Sheriff. I am incredibly lucky to occupy a healthy body. I give thanks for the strength in my arms to carry a toddler into the surf at the beach, and the power in my legs to propel me up mountains on hikes with my family. I feel grateful for the endurance to work a full-time job as well as devote endless hours to eating disorders advocacy.

When I professionally speak and socialize, too, I use humor to combat the ever-present cultural norm of food and body shaming. How? By preemptively declaring myself a "No Body Shaming Zone" at Girls' Nights, work lunches, and everywhere I can. I delight in helping my friends to cease announcing they feel "bad" or "guilty" for eating dessert. And though I am filled with humor about my cultural disobedience nowadays, how I got to this point was not at all funny—terrorizing is more like it. It makes me cherish all the more that I have the energy to approach life with humor and *joie de vivre.*

I invite everyone reading this to ditch the scale and the mindset of restriction. Join me in embracing the freedom of allowing your body and mind to do what they are designed to do. Work toward your own stable weight of "IDGAF"—it's a beautiful, if rebellious and irreverent, place to occupy.

Note from Alli:

As this story states, JD spent decades struggling with the problem of feeling "lesser than" because of her body. As many do, she repeatedly tried to remedy that through weight loss, diet, and exercise, but her weight cycled up and down. Once her daughter developed anorexia nervosa, JD found a most non-traditional way to conquer her own issues. Though her methods came through love, fear, and determination to save her daughter's life, she nonetheless changed her problems into freedom and a better life.

If you're wondering if JD's body image issues somehow caused her daughter's eating disorder, that's human and I get it. "Cause" is complex. Historically, parental influence has often been assumed as the trigger for an eating disorder. This assumption poses problems; it can both get in the way of helpful treatment and be untrue. Notice that all four children were under the same roof, yet one uniquely got an eating disorder.

This story also introduces "negative energy balance," which is a fancy name for what common dieting does (more energy expended than taken in). For a subset of the population, instead of getting anxious when hungry and feeling better when eating, they experience the opposite— feeling calmer and less anxiety when they're empty/emptier. A renowned researcher, Cynthia Bulik, identified this phenomenon in the blog post, "Negative Energy Balance: A Biological Trap for People Prone to Anorexia Nervosa," published by the UNC Center of Excellence for Eating Disorder.[17]

See what I mean by *cause* being complex? Here's a simple answer: no one knows for sure why one person develops an eating disorder and another does not.

The scientific research referenced by the Storyteller about overweight and lifespan refers to the peer-reviewed journal article, "Association of All-cause Mortality with Overweight and Obesity Using Standard Body Mass Index Categories: A Systematic Review and Meta-analysis," by Flegel and colleagues.[18]

Lastly, this story warrants a reminder: advocacy has many forms, from intentional silence to using a bullhorn. What feels most empowering to you, as an advocate, will depend on your unique style in life.

---

[17] Bulik, *Negative Energy Balance: A Biological Trap for People Prone to Anorexia Nervosa*, (2014).
[18] Flegal et al., *Association of All-cause Mortality with Overweight and Obesity Using Standard Body Mass Index Categories: A Systematic Review and Meta-analysis*, (2013).

To My Mom

This is the daughter's side of "The Journey."

Hailey Hershkowitz

AT A YOUNG age, you taught me about self-acceptance. You taught me how to love myself. You taught me that what I saw as my imperfections, others found beautiful; flaws don't have to be ugly. You showed me ways to critically view society's standards of beauty, and that everyone is beautiful in their own way. I never struggled much with body acceptance because you were there to correct and guide me.

Whenever I would put myself down, you would stop me—sometimes mid-sentence—and you'd say, "For every one bad thing about yourself, you have to say two good things about yourself." I now understand why: every time I "affirmed myself," as you called it, I had to both find and say beautiful things about me. Yes, it was a pain while growing up and the last thing I wanted to do. But I think it's a big part of why I never struggled much with my body, why I'm pretty okay with it.

I remember you told me to affirm myself after I stepped on the scale and didn't like my number. Affirming myself carried me through years of dance, cheer, and softball. Even on our family vacations at Lake Powell, it allowed me to run around in a bathing suit with my friends, jumping off cliffs and enjoying myself.

Despite all the fun we have at Lake Powell every year, do you know what I love most? When you and I sit on the back of the boat and fish all day, you bait every hook because I refuse to hook a worm. I have no patience, so I'm constantly reeling it in and then letting it out. But you just sit there for hours because you're *at home*. It's sitting there, not catching fish, being with you. That's what I love the most.

You also taught me that my body is strong and powerful. As my biggest fan and supporter, you told me so all the time. I'm planning to let that strength and power support me during basic training.

What broke my heart was watching the woman, who was nothing short of perfect in my eyes, struggle; you struggled with accepting your own self.

You looked at your own body and single-handedly pointed out each of your flaws, the same flaws that any working woman who birthed two children had. If it weren't you, you would have seen that the supposed flaws only made that woman more beautiful because they told her story. Changes to a body and face naturally happen to any wife and mother, but especially one who puts everyone before herself, one who assures that everyone else is impeccably cared for first.

I watched you offer to take the photo so you wouldn't have to be in it. I was like, "Well that defeats the point of taking the photo if you're not in it." But I could tell that you were uncomfortable, so I didn't push. I still felt let down, though.

I watched you slave in the kitchen almost every day to provide food for your family. Yet when it came time to eat, you were nowhere to be found. And that sucked for me; it made me sad.

I remember you stopped wearing anything that showed your body. You wore really, really oversized clothing. You hid yourself. Before my very eyes, I saw the most beautiful woman in the entire world look at herself in disgust. She didn't realize that people looked at her in awe—I looked at her in awe—and in complete disbelief that a woman that remarkable could envision herself anything less than beautiful.

I think that nowadays you're not worrying as much about what other people think about you, and I love that. You aren't barricading yourself alone anymore, even when you are going through something tough. You planned our first family photo shoot, which was so special to me (and to you too, I think, otherwise, we wouldn't have like 35 shots around the house!). You being *in* the pictures means everything to me. I can see the love among our family members; the camera captured it. Most importantly, I can see your love for yourself—it's in your eyes.

You're already planning the next one with my brother and me in our uniforms. It's super fun to watch you be excited about something you used to feel too self-conscious to do.

I'm proud of you and the work you've done on your journey to self-love. While you made sure that others, including me, had strong foundations of self and body acceptance, you put yourself last. I finally saw you practice what you preach when you began to affirm yourself, and I liked that. You seem to think your biggest flaw is your double chin (which is the same double chin I have at the young age of 18). But I have news for you: Your biggest flaw is not seeing yourself as I see you, in my eyes.

Note from Alli:

Our Storyteller, Hailey, is the daughter of a fellow contributor, Shannon Hershkowitz, and she provides the daughter's view of the story told in "The Journey" of DISCOVERIES. Here, Hailey shares the pain of watching her mother hate her own body. Hailey also expresses her appreciation for her mother having turned her food, weight, and body image problems—which disempowered and disconnected her mom—into empowering and connecting ways of living.

No matter how sly we think we're being in life, people so often see us, noticing what we do and how we feel about ourselves. Commonly, they don't know what to say to us about what they see. They may stay silent, speak "wrong" words, or even avoid us to "not make things worse." I've been around people with eating stresses and disorders for most of, if not my whole life. I've heard those reasons enough to know that all three happen—often and out of care and love.

Hailey mentions her mother's "putting others first," and I notice that many individuals with eating and body image struggles seem have a hard time making themselves a priority. If this sounds like you, too, let's look at this: how are you doing at being able to include moments and activities that enhance your life? Refuel you? Your wellness? Your feeling of contentment? Your sense of balance?

Not so well? That's okay, a lot of us stink at this!

Our self-care goals are often too grand and far away to touch, let alone grasp onto and achieve. Try thinking about what it would take to incorporate a little bit more of what serves and supports you in your life. Any bit can help you to conquer your issues. Go small; do doable.

When we take kinder, more balanced care of ourselves, we tend to depend less on food, dieting, and health-fads to take care of us.

Sweet Ones

Aria Northrop

I AM A 24-year-old preschool teacher who is also in the process of healing from eating and body image issues. I've always been observant of the kiddos. But now that my own disordered eating/eating disorder wrecked some of my life, I especially notice my 3, 4, and 5-year-old munchkins. They already give so much importance to their body image, weight, and worry about "feelings." Year after year, I see it. This is my letter to them, and partly also to myself.

Sweet Ones,

I see you. The girls who stand on step stools to wash their hands and then check their bodies in the bathroom mirror.

I see you. The child who leaves her soft pretzel in her princess lunchbox. She's only eating "healthy" food this week. You have so much growing left to do.

I see you. I know the way your feelings seem to explode out of your body—like the pent-up exhales you are too busy to make while playing. When you're small, your feelings are as big as a grownup's.

I see the way you line your thoughts up before you say them—one after the other, trying to figure out which ones you can speak out loud. Tell me all of them.

The way you hold your thoughts inside you, delicately and fearfully, like you're afraid of the power they will have over you. You are safe here.

It feels like you don't have control over the world around you, like when too many "home days" in a row have made you forget what "crisscross applesauce" means.

You are still worthy. Even when you tell me your dress makes you "look fat," you are still worthy.

Even when you have an outburst because you can't find your water bottle, your lunchbox, your glasses, you are worthy.

On the days you ask me how to love your body, the days I do not have a real answer, you are still worthy.

To the ones who are the smallest in the classroom, and to the ones who ask me if they're "big:" Sometimes, in my home at night, I cry at the beauty you don't yet know you hold.

You are funny, sweet, and daring.

You are so much more than "big."

You are the brightest, fiercest light.

Thank you for shining on me and teaching all your friends how to follow in your footsteps.

Hold onto the things that make you silly, find the things that make you feel safe. You are the bravest ones I know.

Kindly,
Aria

Note from Alli:

This letter reminds us that we were once impressionable and innocent, too. Diet culture can begin influencing us at very young ages—long before we can make well-founded decisions. Research shows that at age 5, many children already express weight-concerns.[19] Then as youngsters developmentally progress during ages 5-8, body dissatisfaction emerges in more mature ways. A study published in 2003 revealed that 59% of the girls and 35% of the boys in that age group wanted to be slimmer.[20] Combine that with an immature but actionable awareness of dieting that also emerges around 5-6,[21, 22] and these children may have years of food and body image stress ahead of them.

When you get down on yourself because dieting or body dissatisfaction feels powerfully influential in your life, keep in mind that you and me have basically been programmed to feel that way. An awareness of media influence (media literacy) can help you to uncover some of that conditioning and assist in your conquering, too.

As this Storyteller observed her little ones with such astuteness and compassion, we may also have been seen that way when we were young. However, parents and teachers can struggle to decipher what's going on with their children and to speak about it in ways that don't overwhelm either party. As a result, sometimes discussions don't happen at

---

[19] Hayes and Tantleff-Dunn, *Am I Too Fat to be a Princess? Examining the Effects of Popular Children's Media on Young Girls' Body Image*, (2010).

[20] Lowes and Tiggemann, *Body Dissatisfaction, Dieting Awareness and the Impact of Parental Influence in Young Children*, (2003).

[21] Dohnt and Tiggemann, *Development of Perceived Body Size and Dieting Awareness in Young Girls*, (2004).

[22] Lowes and Tiggemann, *Body Dissatisfaction, Dieting Awareness and the Impact of Parental Influence in Young Children*, (2003).

all. Then by adulthood, we—grownup you and me—have made whatever limited sense of those early attitudes, actions, interpretations, and experiences.

In each of us, there still lives that little one, precious and pure like those referenced in this Storyteller's letter. As an exercise in self-compassion, I encourage you to consider the following:

- Have a conversation with or write a kind, nurturing letter; make sure you speak from your adult self to your young-you.

- See that young-you through a compassionate lens. What did young-you yearn to hear?

- In your conversation or letter, be an/your ideal, loving, and supportive parent-figure or teacher.

- As with any exercise in compassion, there is little to lose, except perhaps things better off left behind: inaccurate old messages, negative internal voices from the past, long-held but no-longer-serving worldviews, and ultimately, the self-dislike that such old baggage can produce.

She Saved Those

Laura Collins Lyster-Mensh

IT WAS THE giggling. That's how we knew. It wasn't the lack of irritability before meals: that was a slow ebbing over time until the pre-meal clatter was just the expected chaos of a family. It wasn't how much or what was eaten, even though that had been an agonizingly important focus for a long time. It wasn't about food, or eating, or the meal.

It was a giggle. We both heard it, and my husband and I were so startled we both turned our eyes toward our daughter, the giggler. We didn't react, but we caught one another's eyes, and as much as one can shout Hallelujah without seeming to change expression, we both did. She was giggling. Her brother chortled. We all smiled.

There were many other giggles that week, and more every day, but we had been so mirth-free for a long time that I think we had forgotten what they were like. They were sparklers, fireflies, popcorn, and hummingbirds of lighthearted joy.

For months there had been a lack of laughing, of humor except the dark or sarcastic type. Our family, normally ready to laugh and quick to be first on a punchline, had grown serious and generally grim. Jokes had been unseemly and went sour on delivery. When someone among you is tense and unhappy, strained and unshakable, the laughter disappears. And giggles, the hallmark of childhood and the delight of little things, had moved out for a while. We hadn't even noticed. Giggles were the last thing on our minds. Giggles were a luxury we didn't even covet. We would have settled for an unforced smile.

Her eating disorder stole her smile, her laugh, and her giggle. And what a giggle it was. It was the kind of bubbled up silly laugh that drew you closer to share in whatever delight had caused it. Was it a cartoon or a story or a bird outside? Was it the feeling of the sprinkler, or running in the yard with the dog? What game, what new skill, and what friend was she dancing with?

You can't be anxious and giggle. You can't giggle when you're tense. And you can't stop giggling when you hear this kid giggle. It's magic. It was a spell broken.

Of course there were tears, too. It was hard. But she was as brave and as smart as she always was, and still is. She saved the giggles for last as the rest of her unthawed and loosened up. She did not choose to fall down the rabbit hole of an eating disorder, but she saved those giggles inside to come out later. And for all the years since.

Note from Alli:

This Storyteller, Laura, brings up a significant marker that can help you to assess your own quality of life: laughter, which cannot freely flow when you're stressed. Check in and take note. Are you laughing less often because of preoccupations with diet or body image?

People might be missing you. YOU might be missing you. Both are important reasons to persist in seeking your keys to overcoming your food, weight, and body image problems.

Laughter feels good.

Through My 6-Year-Old Daughter's Eyes

Elisheva Dorfman

Admittedly, this is a dramatization, my interpretations of how my daughter experienced me and our past time together. I'm not a mind reader, but as a trained therapist and mother, I know that my daughter struggled to make sense of my actions and attitudes, and then my changes, also. It would be naïve to think she wasn't affected by my choices just because she was too young to talk about it. This is my attempt to give her that voice.

MOMMY USED TO move my hands away if they touched her stomach. I could feel her body go tight. I could see her getting angry, even if it was an accident. I wanted to hug her all over sometimes! But it wasn't allowed.

My legs used to hurt when I walked with her. She went way too fast for me, but she said she needed to "get her heart rate up" or something. She would look at that fitness tracker thing on her wrist to see when it was time to stop walking, and my little brother could *never* get out of his stroller. (He walks *very*, very slow.)

I was sad that we couldn't all eat the same things too. Mommy *only* ate salads. We could only have plain vegetables because she didn't want to make them "fattening." Dinner was no fun at all, to be honest. Mommy was mostly stressed out and angry.

I'm not sure what changed, exactly, but everything is different now. Mommy doesn't diet anymore. She gave it up. She says she wants me to have a healthy relationship with food and with my body. Which I don't completely understand, because she used to insist that dieting was the *same* as "being healthy."

Anyhow, I like the new way much better. I love that now my family eats together at the table, and Mommy can eat the same foods that we are eating. My Mommy even makes spaghetti and cheese sometimes, which is my favorite! She used to make it only with spaghetti squash, but I like real spaghetti better. I'm happy that she figured out how to eat real spaghetti now.

I like that Mommy is calm at dinner. She talks to me and my brother and asks us fun questions about our day. All she used to care about was if I was eating enough, and I'd be in big trouble if I wasn't. But now, she has fun with us! Sometimes my brother throws his food off his highchair, and it makes me laugh. My mommy doesn't get mad anymore when he does that—she laughs and says, "Oh boy..." He also puts food in his hair—icky! (I'm happy I don't have to clean up after him.)

I love how vegetables taste now. My very favorite is to eat red bell peppers with ranch dressing. I love dipping red, yellow, orange, but not green peppers in it. And there are all kinds of other vegetables too! Mommy learned how to cook them all much better. Crispy, salty Brussels sprouts, yum! I like eating my vegetables now.

Mommy used to tell me how much I could eat at meals. She would tell me if I needed to take more bites, and she would tell me if I had to stop eating. Now, Mommy asks me to listen to my belly and my body to know how much to eat. Sometimes I eat too much, but she says, "That's okay! You'll figure it out next time! Listen to your body." Mommy tells me that I am the only one who knows how much food is good for me.

My very favorite is that Mommy doesn't make me go to those long, boring meetings every week anymore. Everyone was nice to me, but then there'd be so many speeches, and weighings, and talking and talking and talking about food. And that was every single Tuesday after school. Now, instead of going there, we go to the library for story time. It's much more fun.

Walks with Mommy are way better now too. She doesn't even *bring* her fitness tracker thing. Now we can stop whenever I feel ready to go back home. And my little brother is allowed to walk around and explore now, no matter how long he takes. She just stands there, letting him wander around like he wants to. (Secretly I think he's happier now too.) I like that Mommy learned how to slow down on our walks. She says she decided that exercise is supposed to be fun, and I like our new way of "exercising" on our walks together!

But the very, very best thing of all is, now Mommy lets me hug her all over. We even went swimming at grandma's house last week, and Mommy came in the *water* in her *bathing suit*. I didn't even know Mommy *had* a bathing suit! It was so much fun splashing and swimming with her. She gave me piggyback rides. I got water in my nose, which I didn't like, but besides that, I had the best time!

I think my Mommy is beautiful. I am so happy that she got rid of the bathroom scale. She used to go on it and cry. I don't know why it made her cry.

My daughter is perceptive—and always thinking, constantly watching. Now 11 years old, I hear her comment about how "different" she finds our family's attitudes about food from some of her friends' homes. Recently, she wondered aloud about some of her close friends at a celebration. She said they had "filled their plates" and "pounded on candy." Then, as if answering her own reflection, she reasoned, "I think it's because their parents don't let them have a lot of treats. You let us have candy, so when we have junk food, we don't start pounding on it." And off she went to play.

I'm SO grateful for realizing that the only way to raise my children with a good relationship to food was to work on and overcome my own stuff. She picks up on so much that I think and do.

Now that my choices are becoming more "healthy" (in thoughtful ways), she has also developed her own personal formula for health. It includes getting enough sleep, eating lots of different kinds of foods, and exercising once a week. Recently she added, "You should not be in front of the screen every day." Out of seemingly nowhere, she included this reference to screen time. Then, I realized that I had logged off social media to spend more quality time with my family.

Our children are always listening, watching, and learning. Our children are always seeing us through their eyes.

Note from Alli:

Elisheva's story challenges us to examine how our actions and attitudes are role modeling for those around us, which we often don't notice. Our unawareness is probably not intentional or conscious. Humans are built to be able to defend ourselves from what we can't (or are not ready to) take in. An example follows.

"Smoking Kid" was an anti-smoking campaign from the Thai Health Promotion Foundation.[23] A hidden camera was used to capture the scenario and natural reactions. With cigarette in hand and as if about to join the unsuspecting smoking adult, the child actor asks, "Can I get a light?" Without fail, each youngster receives a concerned,

---

[23] Thai Health Promotion Foundation, *Smoking Kid*, (2012).

protective response from each adult (e.g., a warning about the dangers of smoking). The child actor then hands the adult a note and exits. The note asks why the adults have forgotten to worry about themselves, too. Every time, the setup seemed to thoughtfully impact—even rattle—each adult.

When you consider our influence on others—including little ones, coworkers, friends, and family—working on conquering dieting, weight, and body image problems in life-benefitting ways might feel even more tempting.

Finding Wellness—You're Not Alone

Celisa Flores

A LACK OF childcare meant that, from the age of four, I'd partake in my mother's stress management efforts. I joined her yoga classes, which probably wasn't meant to evoke a lifelong love. Yet it did.

I remember the instructor highlighting that the practice was designed to relieve the body and mind of stress. Though it was a time before I understood adult "stress," I understood being able to rid yourself of something unwanted—like how the comfort of a hug after a challenging day could make it all go away.

When I grew to adulthood, I wanted to share the joy of yoga and meditation with others. Fortunately, my job at a treatment program had already been incorporating yoga into their evidence-based healing protocols. My employer took me up on my offer to add a trauma-sensitive yoga and meditation focus to the existing program. So after completing an extensive training, I launched into facilitating two yoga groups. One catered to people with dual diagnoses, healing from both a mental health condition and an addiction. The other served people struggling with serious eating and body image issues and diagnoses. The two sets of students could not have responded more differently to yoga and meditation!

The dual-diagnosis group consisted primarily of men who initially resisted joining. But after encouragement from their caseworker, they showed up and "tried it" anyway (often verbally reminding me that they didn't want to be there). For weeks, audible sighs of annoyance filled the room each time we began class with seated observation of our breath and bodies. Then after about a month, participants began to meet any lingering sighs with stern glances, showing me that there had been a shift.

This group reached full capacity each week, and people who had never practiced yoga—some had entered afraid they'd be shamed for not being able to touch their toes— were *hooked.* These students said they felt as if they were taking care of their bodies for the "first time in a long time," and they liked that. Through age-old, simple movements, breath, and stillness, I could see people calming and healing happening. I liked that.

On the other hand, the group with an eating-disorder focus responded *oppositely.* Most of the participants had previously practiced "yoga," and at the outset, they expressed excitement. However, that excitement came to a full and abrupt stop when I announced we would not be practicing a "results-based," "calorie burning" activity.

We then spent significant time discussing the concepts of joyful movement, body nurturing, and self-care practices. But these students could not seem to comprehend or agree that forms of yoga—or any form of movement, for that matter—could have a purpose other than caloric burn. I remember one student loudly expressing that this form of yoga and meditation sounded like a "waste of time." The other students emphatically nodded in agreement.

Despite their protests, I offered the class I'd been employed to teach. My style of instruction has typically focused on breathing, moving gently, and learning the needs of your body so you can respect them. For example, we practiced yogic breathing in soothing, low light. The pace offered participants space for stillness and quiet self-reflection, which most filled with restless fidgeting, tears, or heavy sobs instead. Some called the silent meditations "grueling." Others titled their tears as "tears of boredom." Some participants got up and left mid-class (repeatedly). I remember one student even disrupted the start of class by practicing handstands!

As an instructor, I felt uncomfortable, sometimes even guilty. There I was, giving people something that seemed like bad-tasting medicine to them. My intentions were to *help*, not upset them.

Believing in the ancient practices, I persisted. And slowly, glimpses of progress happened, like a few deep breaths, a decrease in collective sobs, or a slight smile during silent meditation. The students were beginning to come into the practice, meaning their energy was starting to settle. When you can be with yourself in a neutral way, you can learn about what you like and what you want to change.

Months into running this group, one person said, "I'm sad that it took me this long to sit with myself." (YES! *Someone* had experienced the magic and wonder I had experienced in yoga as a child.) From here, we'll call her "Jessica" for confidentiality purposes.

Thrilled about the breakthrough, I invited a conversation about her experience—the shift from "battle" mentality (the mind fighting with stillness and quiet) to viewing yoga and meditation as opportunities for inquiry and observation—both of which can provide a person with the freedom to respond from a place of awareness, rather than react from a place of urgency or fear. By the time Jessica's treatment at the facility ended, she no longer viewed herself as being victimized by her thoughts. Instead, yoga and meditation had become places where she felt empowered to explore her own experience. And Jessica was not alone in this transformation.

After she completed her program, she and I stayed in contact through the center's different alumni groups. I've learned that Jessica has maintained her daily yoga and meditation practices. She no longer goes to yoga classes that emphasize results, caloric burn, or even that have mirrors. Her practice of yoga with meditation and breathwork typically occurs at home, alone. She told me that she sometimes discusses her observations with friends or her therapist, but mostly feels free to observe without the need to "do" anything. She has learned to be fine with "being."

Contrary to some understandings, in any meditation practice, the state of being does not mean apathy. It simply means that we can rest confidently in the awareness that we have the fortitude to be all right no matter what. We may question, and then choose whether or not to enlist our precious resources, such as asking for support, help, and guidance.

As she experienced the challenges of both life and healing from her eating disorder, Jessica said that the gentle inquiry helped her find "calm in the storm," keeping her centered on her ability to come back to peace, internally, even when things felt chaotic externally. Jessica began to trust herself and her observations.

The experiences I have shared here are not isolated to people with official eating disorders or dual diagnoses. I see people shift like this in my studio practice too—people probably similar to those reading this book.

Many of us struggle to allow our thoughts to *be* with us and not judged by us. This is the challenge and growth of Mindfulness meditation and yoga. In moments of stillness, it can feel as if the brain is screaming, the body is the enemy, and another rigid program yells that it's the fix for your problems. In the silence, though, people often find other options—options that enrich their lives either in lieu of (or at least in addition to) harsher practices. Change usually happens slowly, and eventually, some choose to add more self-compassion to their coping toolboxes.

We all have the power to find peace in our internal experience, even if only briefly. That flicker of a different, calmer experience can make all the difference. We all have the power to rid ourselves of something unwanted. Maybe yoga and meditation can help to support your exploration of how you might rid yourself of extra pain and worry in your life—especially if related to food, weight, and body image issues.

As an instructor, I have had 12 beautiful years thus far of witnessing the transformative power in "being" instead of urgently "doing." As a participant since age four, yoga has felt like a "wellness-practice" in my life. I encourage you to find your wellness practices. They are out there— possibly right here.

Note from Alli:

This Storyteller, Celisa, and I want readers to have resources on the possible benefits of yoga. She provided this: for evidence-based information about yoga and its many applications, the International Journal of Yoga (ijoy.org.in.)[24] now publishes quarterly peer-reviewed articles.

---

[24] International Journal of Yoga

Personally, I wrestle with implying that yoga and meditation are not "traditional" approaches for overcoming issues. The practices of both are quite old, are revered by many, and have years of evidence supporting their benefits. Nonetheless, these gentle options are still probably infrequently recommended when compared with the harsher, more immediate, and directive approaches, such as increasing rigidity around diet and exercise to "battle the bulge" or "win the war" with food, weight, willpower, whatever.

Seriously, how long can anyone withstand being in active combat with self? Yoga and meditation might help you to discover, or become part of, your own wellness practices that can be maintained long-term.

To Get Through All of It

This story is my mom's side of
"Alli's Clumsy Conquering—My Story Leading to
this Book"

Patricia R. Spotts

I DON'T KNOW anyone else who raised three children and went through menopause with a brain tumor the size of a grapefruit. Little did I or anyone else recognize that I was paddling through my busy life with one oar or wonder whether I would've been a better mom without the brain tumor. But in the end, there was enough love to get us through all of it.

On July 2, 1971, my husband and I went into the hospital thinking our baby would be named Jeffery, joining brothers, John and Jim. After an easy-peasy delivery, it was a surprise and thrill to welcome a baby girl into our family. Dad cried tears of joy. When the nurse put her on her tummy in the baby nursery, she fought to lift her head—a foretelling of what was to come!

Needing to name our daughter to leave the hospital and inspired by the family name, Alice, we decided on "Allison." From then on, by my side, "Alli" went everywhere with the family. With an easy-going and happy nature, she was our "frosting on the cake."

One day, when Alli was about two-and-a-half, I was walking past her room. She was looking at herself in a full-length mirror, nothing too weird about that. "Am I pretty, Mama?" she asked me. I soothed her, but what struck me was, she had her nose pressed against the mirror (literally flattened), her eyes less than an inch from the glass. Why so close? And then I recalled, when the kids would turn off the television after watching *I Love Lucy*, Alli would say, "Lucy is all through talking." Just talking? I put these two oddities together and decided to have her vision checked.

An evaluation from a pediatric ophthalmologist revealed that our Alli had complex vision problems that required her to wear glasses immediately. The thick, heavy double lenses looked as if they were made from Coca-Cola bottles. Her dad and I worried they would hold her back, but nothing did. In her preschool and elementary school years, she spent her time earning good grades, writing adorable scripts for puppet plays, performing in little talent shows, playing with her Barbie dolls, and watching her brothers play baseball. (Sports were not for Alli as her vision issues made it impossible to track a ball.)

ALLI **SPOTTS-DE LAZZER**

By the time she had reached 6th grade, her eyes had improved so much that she needed glasses only for reading. She began to garner compliments from people on her beauty, even approaching her with modeling opportunities. With the new attention Alli was receiving, her confidence soared. Our once-bookworm joined all sorts of afterschool activities.

That Alli was lovely, talented, and full of enthusiasm did not mean she was immune to bullying. In seventh grade at a charity walk, a few of her classmates surrounded Alli and her friend. They doused them with water, spat on them, and said nasty things about Alli.

It was shortly after this incident, I noticed Alli had odd habits with her food—and our food too. Her father would want some peanut butter, and he'd find it was dry because Alli had drained all the oil from it. She loved spaghetti, but she began to push it around the plate until it landed on the floor where the dogs would happily clean up for her. She started buying cereal with her allowance and then hiding it in her room, so her brothers would not touch it. If anyone prepared food for her, she'd get prickly. It is now more than 36 years ago for me, and I still recall her daily diet of broccoli, a bagel and cream cheese (every once in a while), and her hoarded cereal.

Her food complications totally confused me, and when I challenged her to eat (or eat more), it made a bad situation worse. I pretended I didn't notice her struggle because I didn't want her feeling judged. I would congratulate her for eating broccoli, thinking at least it had some healthiness to it. The only information I had about eating disorders was what I understood from recent news— that Karen Carpenter died from a heart problem caused by something called *anorexia*, which involved not eating enough. I refused to believe that could happen to Alli.

One year, our annual family vacation to Mexico was so stressful. Alli packed her record player and a few dance records and insisted on bringing them with us. She aerobicized upstairs in her bedroom for hours and barely ate. When she ran out of sugarless gum, she behaved as if regular gum was toxic. We spent hours walking and searching stores in town for sugarless gum. Adding to the distress of the trip, Alli's brother pointed out her protruding vertebrae when we sat behind her at the beach. Still, no one in the family "got it."

Once I came home and found Alli with a scarlet red face, sweaty, and breathless. She had wrapped her body in cling wrap, put on a sweat suit, and swaddled a beach towel around her shoulders. She had been on our exercise bike pedaling for hours. OMG! Now an exercise problem, too? I knew something was very wrong, and I tried to get help from her doctor, but he recommended I shouldn't talk about her eating habits in front of her. So I didn't. Our HMO then paired her with a therapist who seemed as helpful as a tit on a boar, and I suspect that Alli put up with her and said what she thought the therapist wanted to hear.

I knew the anorexia was something very real, but that didn't mean I knew how to handle it. Nobody knew much about eating disorders in the eighties. I couldn't control it, and the behaviors were baffling—it was making Alli depressed, angry, unpredictable, and tense. At the time, the best I could do was to make sure Alli knew she was loved and felt secure at home, and I tried to do that.

As all this all happened, I was also coping with two teenage boys, a part-time job, a stressed marriage, and my own struggle. My behavior was erratic and my physical health in decline from that undiagnosed brain tumor. Through all this, Alli and I became codependent on one another, and I felt she was the only friend I had. I think we felt "safe" with one another. I not only loved her, I needed her.

Since therapy seemed ineffective and she had been labeled as having an eating disorder, we sent her to an eating disorder treatment program. She attended an outpatient clinic at a hospital downtown, which greatly upset her. She got angry at her father and me about missing after school activities. Doors slammed, and she shouted at us. During treatment, she got even more hostile and volatile.

Contrary to her usual high performance, she didn't do well in treatment. It was recommended that she be put into an in-hospital care program, which we could not afford. Our insurance did not cover eating disorder illnesses. She discontinued the program and seemed to calm down. Physically, she was slim, but not as alarmingly so. We figured she was doing better, even though I could tell she still hated to come to the dinner table.

In June of 1989, my health problems ended shortly after Alli's graduation from high school—my brain tumor was removed! Life was great for me again, and the family had to adjust to a new, euphoric mother and wife. I was fortunate and will always be grateful I recovered.

Alli went to college, where she was fun to be with and always seemed up for having a good time. Her dad and I thoroughly enjoyed her college years. When appropriate, she invited us to attend her activities. She seemed to be both thriving and blossoming. As with high school, Alli maintained very good grades in college, graduating with honors.

Looking back, her dieting and eating disorders were undoubtedly more difficult for Alli than they were for us. Life was hard for her, but she was adept at hiding her struggles. Her personality was prickly around food, sure, but she never got mad at Dad and me, except during her brief time in treatment at the eating disorder clinic.

When Alli announced one day that, for more than 20 years, eating issues and weight had been the primary focus of her life and her memories, I was shocked. She explained that she'd met a really special guy and wanted to remember building a life with him. She said that Dad and I were getting older, and she wanted real memories with us, too. So, in her persistent and organized Alli-way, she dug into changing. A chart went up where she'd put a star on each day she got through without engaging in destructive behaviors.

I was so used to her food issues that it confused me the first time she took a couple bites of dessert and put her fork down. There was no negative or anxious energy. No prickly. No bitchy. I couldn't help but ask how she could do that. Two bites of chocolate is impossible for me because I love it so much. She said, "I'm done. I'm happy." I felt skeptical. Was she deceiving both herself and me again?

Then one Thanksgiving, a few years after Alli committed to dealing with her eating issues, we sat down for this holiday meal. Our family loved to welcome friends and people who were far from home or had nowhere to go, so the celebration was well attended. Suddenly, we all heard a huge cracking sound. Then CRASH! The chair Alli had been sitting on broke and smashed to the ground with her in it. One of the guests who knew nothing of Alli's history or struggles yelled, "FATTY!" and proceeded to crack himself up. He laughed alone. The rest of us didn't make a move or a sound.

I was sure the prickly old Alli (for whom *every* celebration was ruined by the food angst caused by her stress from her eating struggles) was going to crawl up from the floor and not be pleasant. Instead, I heard a deep belly laugh spilling up and over the table. The rest of the family broke into nervous laughter as it dawned on us: our high-spirited, full-of-life Alli was back. She hadn't been able to laugh *at* herself or silly things that happened in her life for a long, long time.

If I had it to do over, I'd do a lot of it differently. Sometimes I feel guilty. I didn't have a proper focus because

I was sick, too. And there wasn't the information and help available then that there is now. Thankfully, we got to know and like each other all over again, we are both well today, and there was enough love to get us through all of it.

Note from Alli:

This is my mom's experience of my eating, weight, and body image issues, and I can imagine this wasn't easy for her to revisit. Few of us are trained in what to do when problematic eating or body issues emerge from self or others. That said, if you feel confused, curious, or regretful about something related to those issues, please allow the uncomfortable emotions to stay with you. Why? They can help fuel you to take beneficial action.

If you've experienced furniture giving out from under you, this story might have brought up feelings for you. Diet culture makes it seem okay to comment and make fun of weight-related incidents without recognizing the harm. I was not doing that here; my response to shock is often laughter, and suddenly finding myself on the floor jolted me into my normal reaction of unbridled giggles.

Also, contrary to this story, sometimes love is not enough to get people through their battles with eating, dieting, body image, or eating disorders. If the struggle has taken over the person and they're stuck in their obsessive or driven ways, they'll often push people away, isolate, put loved ones "on eggshells," or keep their friends and family at a distance. Not all relationships will survive the strains of these stresses. In addition, sometimes the body will become damaged, weak, or even give out. I know caring people—parental figures, spouses, partners, and friends—who ooze love, but either their person is not in the relationship with them (e.g., distanced or broken up), or their loved one's body did not withstand the driven-dieting, restriction, malnutrition, purging, or exercise.

Finally, readers, about the cling wrap thing: NO! It can be dangerous to your health AND is ineffective for real weight loss. I didn't know those warnings (and probably wouldn't have cared back then). Now *you* know. Don't do it.

EPILOGUE

IN A TIDY-ISH WRAPPER: THE WRAP UP

BECAUSE THE TITLE refers to "conquering" dieting, weight, and body image issues, you might have expected this book to give you strategies to strengthen your willpower or teach you how to become stricter with—"control"—your diet, exercise, and health rules. Instead, these stories offered you more flexible, compassionate-but-real skills found through others' life experiences. Each narrative reveals at least one shift from eating, weight, and body image problems to life-enriching perspectives and practices.

Though the Storytellers depicted here are as diverse as their experiences, commonalities can be found in their discoveries, insights, and connections related to science, behaviors, beliefs, and lifestyle.

Science

- Restricting or dieting can set us up for bingeing.

- Biology plays a profound role in influencing each of our shapes and sizes.

- Unnatural eating and weight loss practices typically come with unwanted consequences.

- Weight does not equal, nor can it singularly measure, health.

Behaviors and beliefs

- Eating and diet can become intertwined with a sense of morality. What you eat does not make you a good or bad human being.

- A person may not know they have an eating disorder. They may be convinced that their beliefs and actions are in service of their health and/or weight.

- Irregular eating behaviors, purging, and extreme exercise practices can negatively affect your physical, medical, mood, and cognitive wellness. These stories pointed out only some of the possible consequences. Nearly every organ system in the body can undergo harm.

- Many think they'll feel good enough, fit in, or be accepted once they reach a particular size, shape, or health status. In my experience, the problem usually goes deeper than this.

Lifestyle

- Movement that you enjoy is usually sustainable; "I have to" exercise, on the other hand, is most often not.

- Mindfulness can help us connect with our natural, internal guides.

- Questioning your thoughts and beliefs about body and dietary intake can help correct inaccuracies.

- Identifying, accepting, and working through feelings can be a part of healing from eating and body problems.

- Food, weight, and body issues can distract you from what genuinely needs attention, care, or change.

- Gaining a full and balanced existence might come from giving up traditional dieting, weight loss, or exercise programs.

- Life without—or with less of a focus on—dieting, weight, and body image can be pretty darn great.

If these takeaways may have seemed uncommon, rebellious, or even wrong to you, I understand. Initially, I felt the same way. Yet science and experience both support these viable points. Traditional messaging ("Diet better and exercise more") is not necessarily *the way* to conquer your issues.

Whether you desire full freedom from your food, weight, and body battles or to have a tad less torment, "conquering" tends to be a process that includes individualized elements and can take time to achieve. Yet one thing is for certain: change takes active participation from you. I encourage you to keep going. Find your way to your meaningFULL life, one freer of food and body image struggles.

To further explore paths and principles mentioned in these pages, check out the Resources section. There are many potentially beneficial options out there to support you. For example, when discussing this book with friends and colleagues, I was reminded that people find their desired level of conquering through various ways, sometimes including strong support systems, faith, evidence-based treatments, therapists, registered dietitians, consultants, coaches, medical doctors, specialized treatment programs, self-help aids, support groups, Chinese medicine, 12-step recovery programs, and addiction approaches. I do not deem the philosophies and concepts in this book as the *only* valuable modes for all people, since that could limit *your* process.

Please *thoroughly* research anything you might try for overcoming your eating, weight, and body image stresses, and don't trust every source. Information about food, diet, and health tends to be varied, evolving, and sometimes controversial or even false. Bad information is out there, some of it dressed up in trappings that can appear official or scholarly. Data and advice will likely serve best when both align with your goals, core values, and good science. If something you try is safe, life-enhancing, and not punishing, you'll probably have a better chance of maintaining it long-term.

As many of these stories demonstrated, the difference between someone uber-focused on managing their food and body size versus someone with a clinical eating disorder can seem unclear—especially to the person. If you feel concerned about yourself or someone you love, a professional trained in eating disorders can usually help tease out the diagnostic aspects and offer you information. Rest assured, though, that any problem labeled or diagnosis received is only one of the many parts of any human being. No one *is* their label(s); each of us is a person with multiple dimensions.

WARNING: almost anyone can state they "specialize" in eating disorders, weight, and body issues. I encourage you to vet a professional's competence and expertise. Ask questions. Assess if they're a supportive and a potentially effective match. Inquiries might include:

- What is your training and experience specifically in eating disorders, disordered eating, dieting, weight, and body image issues?

- When and what was the last conference or continuing education course you attended that focused on eating disorders/eating, body image, or weight issues?

- What is your approach to helping me with my dieting, weight, and body image issues? *If you want to incorporate weight-neutrality/weight-inclusivity, Health At Every Size® principles, Intuitive Eating, mindful eating, etc. in your pursuit of health, you'll want to ask if the professional utilizes these approaches.*

Because it's difficult to gauge what's "enough" to feel assured your provider is proficient, here's an idea: consider their hours of training, education, and experience in relationship to your own familiarity with these topics. I imagine that you want someone with significant knowledge that you might eventually trust. There are competent certified, "CED," and non-certified providers. I wish that screening practitioners was a more straightforward, easier task for you.

Be aware that many potential helpers will align with a one-size-fits-all weight-focused mentality that favors thin. This can be due to a personal bias, training, background, or something else. But a one-size approach can miss out on honoring diverse bodies and overlook important life-factors that figure into overall wellness.

Focusing on BMI, weight, and numbers as the main yardsticks of health can *intensify* food, weight, and body image issues. So, for a more accurate measure of your whole health, please consider adding personal, well-rounded markers. Some Storytellers included social connectedness, a balanced life, satisfying physical activity, and self-compassion in their health snapshots. To clarify yours, try asking yourself:

- What do health and wellness mean to me?

- Understanding that my body, mind, and metabolism are uniquely mine, what do I need to achieve the most effective and contented version of me?

Once you get an inkling of your answers to these questions, you'll be better able to find who or what feels aligned with your goals.

I want to acknowledge that for some, *complete* freedom from restriction or food eliminations may not be advised or possible due to food allergies and medical conditions such as Crohn's disease, diabetes, cardiovascular disease, celiac disease, and others. If this is you, I encourage you to seek a trained medical or nutritional professional to help you navigate your path. Someone who is well versed in a non-diet, weight-neutral/weight-inclusive approach may prove both healthful and helpful.

In Conclusion, "Why the Heck Not?"

If eating, weight, and body image issues are getting in the way of living a more satisfying existence, why not try something different? The discoveries, insights, connections, and hope offered in this book provide powerful keys to help you unlock more of what you want—a meaningful life with fewer to no stresses over food, dieting, shape, size, and body image.

What have you got to lose? Our weight-focused and "health"-driven cultures with their ensuing fad diets, newest weight-loss trends, and superfood crazes will patiently wait for you. Mega businesses depend on *your* dissatisfaction with yourself for *their* profit. Besides, if freedom doesn't work for you, you can always go back to whatever you were doing.

We get one life to make as healthy, connected, and meaningful as we want. I know firsthand as both a professional and someone who recovered from dieting and eating disorders, change can happen, and there is hope.

What might your meaningFULL life look and feel like?

May you begin it today.

ABOUT OUR STORYTELLERS

Thank you to our contributors for sharing their stories.

Angelica. Female. World traveler. Flawed human. Working on compassion for self and others daily.

Anonymous ("My Body Wasn't the Enemy"). After a 15-year struggle with food/weight, this mid-30's city girl, wife, mother, sister, and friend received life-changing treatment. She has never looked back.

Anonymous ("Never Going to be Perfect"). Her various incarnations in this life have been as a Broadway dancer, singer, business owner, and mother. She started dancing at the age of five and hasn't stopped. Her interpersonal superpowers have been used to represent directors and composers for commercials. Her son continues to be her greatest teacher.

Anonymous ("Take the Body I'm Giving You"). Anonymous is a spiritual warrior for sisterhood. She loves her husband, her family, and the Divine. She values compassion, courage, and wit. Her message to others is "Be kind, but be kind to yourself FIRST."

Anonymous ("What a Trip!") was born and raised in Colorado and now lives with her wife and dog in California. She is an acupuncturist and herbalist who loves to travel, read, hike, practice tai chi, and play dodgeball.

Anonymous ("What I Took for Granted"). She enjoys telling stories to music. She loves her husband, family, animals, and career. Message to readers: don't worry if you don't nail the right career on the first try. You'll be amazed how things come together in time.

Billy Blanks Jr. is a fitness expert known for creating feel-good fitness programs that make movement and exercise fun. Though he has starred on stage, appeared on television, choreographed for celebrities, and directed high profile shows, he is most proud of being Elijah's father.

Elisheva Dorfman is a mom to two children. She has her master's degree in psychology and works as a psychotherapist. She loves to hike and bake. Without dieting, she lives a happier and healthier life. Her goal is to raise children who love themselves, others, all foods, and their bodies.

Aaron Flores is a registered dietitian living in Los Angeles, CA. He is married and is a father to boy and girl twins. When he's not at work, he enjoys golfing, writing, and spending time with his friends arguing which is really the best *Star Wars* film ever.

Celisa Flores is a lifelong student in the realms of yoga, meditation, motherhood, breathwork, and psychology with experiential and formal training. Dr. Flores's message to others: "Your growth is never too delicate to withstand pruning."

Veronica Garcia. Woman proud of her Mexican heritage, 45 years lived so far. Mother of two. Grandmother of four. One of five siblings. College educated. Put herself through grad school. Independent. Strong. Loving.

Jaynie M. Goldberg is a wife, mother, businesswoman, boss, and friend. She enjoys serving through volunteer work that feels meaningful. She adores her husband and their three children, two boys and a girl. She strives to be present in her kids' lives and cherishes being there for all their "firsts."

Beau-Haim Harang is a 40-year-old, happily married man with many accomplishments professionally. His personal life was sometimes beautiful and other times devastating. He enjoys art, music, creating, and helping people. "To my Joao, Jack, Mum, Georgia, family, and God, I love you. Michel, thank you for saving my life."

Hailey Hershkowitz. Daughter. Sister. Airman. Friend.

Shannon Hershkowitz. World traveler who shares her greatest adventure to self-acceptance.

Laura James is a sorcerer of social services, an adventurer, an aspiring on-key singer, a first-time-golfer, a one-time paddleboarder, a repeat aerobics class taker, and a try-just-about-anything-once person. She values integrity, being the wife and beloved of Jake, and the proud mom of Violet.

Staci Lawrence, an actress, dancer, and comedienne, was born and raised outside Detroit. Graduating Summa Cum Laude, she studied Theatre at Western Michigan University and toured Greece performing. Staci co-founded Flash Mob America, the world's first flash mob production company. Her husband and two children are her greatest joys in life.

Laura Collins Lyster-Mensh, M.S., is a writer who became an activist for improved eating-disorder treatment after the recovery of her teen daughter from anorexia. She has written two books on eating disorders, *Eating With Your Anorexic* and *Throwing Starfish Across the Sea.* She is the Executive Director of F.E.A.S.T., a nonprofit serving families around the world who support a loved one with an eating disorder.

Aurora Miceli never quite felt like she fit in growing up. She was quirky, different—even asked by a school to not return because it wasn't a good fit. She shares, "After recently turning my age, I'm telling my truths. I'm comfortable in my own skin and loving every minute of it."

Aria Northrop is currently a preschool teacher with a helper's heart. She's passionate, supportive, enthusiastic, loving, and inspired by learning about psychology. Her future is unknown—she's in her early 20's. What is for sure is this: she is working on freedom from eating disorders, which have been the opposite of freedom.

JD Ouellette is a professional educator, activist, wife, mother, and grandmother. She writes, speaks, and presents on eating disorders. Ouellette also provides peer support and is passionate about using a social justice filter in her work. At 55, she is comfortable in her own skin and wants the same for all.

Patricia R. Spotts. Wife, mother, retired schoolteacher, and participant in Church activities.

RESOURCES

Here is a short list of accessible resources. Please note that it is wholly your responsibility to review and vet for fit, helpfulness, your feeling of safety, etc. No sponsorship or formal endorsement existed between the author and these outlets at the time this book was composed. This list is offered exclusively as leads for readers to explore when seeking potential health and quality of life improvements. *Listed in alphabetical order.*

Academy for Eating Disorders (AED)

"The Academy for Eating Disorders is a global professional association committed to leadership in eating disorders research, education, treatment, and prevention."

www.aedweb.org

Be Nourished

"Informed by shame resilience theory, social justice movements, and self-compassion while working from the principles of Intuitive Eating and Health At Every Size®, Be Nourished offers programs, workshops, retreats, and e-courses for individuals looking to reclaim Body Trust®."

www.benourished.org

Dieting, Stress and Health (DiSH) Lab

"The DiSH Lab at UCLA studies the intersection between eating, not eating (dieting), stress, and health. We study how emotions affect eating, but also how eating affects emotions. We also study how these emotion-eating links contribute to health, illness, and aging."

http://www.dishlab.org/

Ellyn Satter Institute

"Ellyn Satter has devoted her long career to uplifting the mealtime experience. She teaches parents how to transform family meals into joyful, healthful, struggle-free events, free from drama and conflict. She teaches individuals with weight issues how to release themselves from the grip of guilt and shame in their relationship with food."

https://www.ellynsatterinstitute.org

F.E.A.S.T. (Families Empowered And Supporting Treatment for Eating Disorders)

The global organization of and serving parents and caregivers around the world. "We are here to help you understand your son or daughter's eating disorder, support you in helping them get appropriate treatment, and get you the information you need to help them recover and thrive."

https://www.feast-ed.org/

Health At Every Size® (HAES)®

"Health At Every Size principles help us advance social justice, create an inclusive and respectful community, and support people of all sizes in finding compassionate ways to take care of themselves." Health At Every Size® and HAES® are registered trademarks of the Association for Size Diversity and Health and used with permission.

www.haescommunity.com

International Association of Eating Disorders Professionals (iaedp™)

Organization for multidisciplinary treatment professionals that "offers a highly respected certification process for those who wish to receive specialized credentials in their work with people with eating disorders."

www.iaedp.com

Intuitive Eating

"Intuitive Eating is a self-care eating framework, which integrates instinct, emotion, and rational thought and was created by two dietitians, Evelyn Tribole and Elyse Resch in 1995. This book is in its 4th edition."

www.intuitiveeating.org

National Association for Anorexia Nervosa and Associated Disorders (ANAD)

"ANAD is the oldest organization aimed at fighting eating disorders in the United States. ANAD assists people struggling with eating disorders and also provides resources for families, schools and the eating disorder community."

www.anad.org

National Eating Disorders Association (NEDA)

NEDA is "the largest nonprofit organization dedicated to supporting individuals and families affected by eating disorders. NEDA supports individuals and families affected by eating disorders, and serves as a catalyst for prevention, cures, and access to quality care."

www.nationaleatingdisorders.org

Self-Compassion (website) by Dr. Kristin Neff

Though this website is not diet specific, "self-compassion" can be a necessary inner quality. According to Dr. Neff, "Having compassion for oneself is really no different than having compassion for others."

www.selfcompassion.org

UCLA Mindful Awareness Research Center

This webpage contains "an introduction to mindfulness meditation that you can practice on your own." Guided meditations are currently made available for download at no cost. *Recorded by UCLA MARC's Director of Mindfulness Education, Diana Winston.*

https://www.uclahealth.org/marc/mindful-meditations

ACKNOWLEDGMENTS

THOUGH I AM the author of *MeaningFULL*, this could only have happened through community. To all who were involved in making this book possible, I send a heartfelt thank you.

Unsolicited Press, I feel grateful for your partnership. Thank you for believing in this book.

My husband, Michael, oh my goodness, you are a patient and loving man—and a fab storyteller. Mom, you are still a rock star with English and a terrific canary in the coalmine. John, Sonia, and Jim, thank you for your tireless patience and help. Dad, Bek, and Paul—you supported, too! Betsy, thanks for un-retiring your talent. Connie Call, my therapist, you are a part of who I've become.

Since this began around three years ago, I've kept an ongoing list of colleagues, friends, acquaintances, and strangers who were blessings along the way. At the start, I had limited knowledge of how to curate this kind of book, and there has been a lot of learning, trial, and error. Ranging anywhere from answering a "quick question" to test reading the entire book and giving feedback, thank you to these beautiful souls: Emily Aaronson, Elisabeth Abbott, Karen Adair, Lauren Anton, Carrie Arnold, Jessica Barker, Jilly Becerra, Carolyn Becker, Barbara Benouilid, Lynne Biehl, Michele C. Blake, Cindy Bouchard, Shelita Burke,

Esther Bursztyn, Regan Carrington, Ruth Carter, Devon Cole, Amy Cook, Leila Costa, Lisa Dalesandro, Maureen Dall, Jennifer Detisch, Lori DiCostanzo, Suzanne Dooley-Hash, Allison Donovan, Elisheva Dorfman, Barbara Eberhard, Patty Everett, Max Fierstein, Lana Ford, Jonna Fries, Marise Frietas, Beau-Haim Harang, Beth Harrell, Camissa Hill, Laura James, Natalie Janji, Jenny Januszewski, Leslie Kaplan, Raduca Kaplan, Pamela Keel, Michael Klein, Katie-Lily Lambert, Kathleen MacDonald, Christine Maher, Norah McIntire, Grace Medina, Joy Morales-Bartlett, Darren Moran, Michelle Nickel, JD Ouellette, Molly Paige, Sara Detisch Peck, Josie Perrone, Mira Reverente, Kristen Rose, Shira Rosenbluth, Samantha Scruggs, Jeff Slattery, Michelle Smith, Lindsay Stuart, Mara Tyler, Caroline Watson, and June Westerfield. To Robyn Caruso, Lauren Muhlheim, and Laura Westmoreland, I deeply respect your passion for protecting people, and I appreciate your enduring support of my spirited ways. Barbara De Santis, you patiently taught me what I needed to do. Nadyja Von Ebers, glad to have found you. Robert "Bob" Nickel, you have been a tremendous help! Our Facebook grammar conversations led me back to your incredible talent and heart. And to the beyond-patient Storytellers—thank you for not killing me, even if you might have wanted to with my eternal changes. For anyone I missed mentioning, I'm so sorry! You *are* appreciated.

Funny moment... One day I was being hard on myself in a conversation with Mom. She says, "I'm going to quit reading these if you're not nicer to me." I say, "I'm being hard on myself." She says, "I know. You're just awful to yourself! I'm going to quit if you're not nicer." This book is a lot about self-compassion, so I have laughed at the irony of this often. #EternalGrowth

CONCEPTS AND CLARIFIED TERMS

PEOPLE WHO STRUGGLE with eating and body issues often have practices and attitudes that span from slightly to severely disruptive to their lives. What's the difference between someone who's "always on a diet" and has body dislike versus someone with a clinical eating disorder? It depends. Here's a quick and easy generalization that might help you to conceptualize: a person with an eating disorder seems unable to "normally" eat. Their *choices* about food and exercise become "*I have to*" or "*I must*;" they cannot *not* do what they feel they need to do.

Highlights of important concepts and terms follow (indicated by **bolded**).[25]

- If someone has an **eating disorder**, it means they have a diagnosable psychological illness. People may not know they have an eating disorder; they may think they are simply dieting and being healthy.

- A person who regularly takes actions to get thinner such as refusing to eat, restricting intake, etc.; intensely fears gaining weight; and can't see their body accurately might match with an **anorexia nervosa** diagnosis. We now know that people at

---

[25] These descriptions are not intended or sufficient for diagnosis. Please allow a professional to do that.

higher weights, not just extremely low, can develop this disorder.

- A person who regularly **binges** (eats a lot of food in a certain period of time and feels out of control while doing it); tries to get rid of the calories by **purging** (emptying body of food consumed), exercising, fasting, or other methods; and tends to morally judge themself as a good/bad person by their body size/weight might correspond with a **bulimia nervosa** diagnosis.

- A person who regularly binges; feels tremendous guilt, sadness, or stress about it; and doesn't necessarily try to negate the calories might go with a **binge-eating disorder** diagnosis.

- A person who has either some of the mentioned or related attitudes and behaviors—enough to cause distress—may gain a diagnosis of **Other Specified/Unspecified Feeding and Eating Disorders (OSFED/UFED)**.

- Though not clear even in the professional world, key differences between **OSFED/UFED** and **"normal dieting"** or the other diagnoses depend on a few things. These can include the level of distress the person experiences, how much the symptoms affect their daily life, or the ease of stopping the behaviors/modifying the attitudes.

Those are my interpretations of select features of some of the disorders that fall under the main category, **Feeding and**

Eating Disorders,[26] in the Diagnostic and Statistical Manual-5, the sourcebook of mental health diagnoses. If you're interested in detailed, user-friendly information on these and related topics, the Resources section in this book provides weblinks to U.S.-based and international organizations.

---

[26] American Psychiatric Association, *Diagnostic and Statistical Manual of Mental Disorders (5th ed.),* (2013).

INDEX

BIBLIOGRAPHY

"The U.S. Weight Loss & Diet Control Market." *Market Research*, Marketdata LLC., 3 May 2017, www.marketresearch.com/Marketdata-Enterprises-Inc-v416/Weight-Loss-Diet-Control-10825677/.

Bulik, Cynthia. "Negative Energy Balance: A Biological Trap for People Prone to Anorexia Nervosa." *Exchanges*, UNC Center of Excellence for Eating Disorders, 1 Dec. 2014, uncexchanges.org/2014/12/01/negative-energy-balance-a-biological-trap-for-people-prone-to-anorexia-nervosa/.

Costin, Carolyn. "About Carolyn Costin." *Carolyn Costin*, 2018, www.carolyn-costin.com/about.

Devlin, Keith. "Top 10 Reasons Why The BMI Is Bogus." *NPR*, NPR, 4 July 2009, www.npr.org/templates/story/story.php?storyId=106268439.

Diagnostic and Statistical Manual of Mental Disorders (5th Ed), American Psychiatric Association, 2013, pp. 329–354.

Dohnt, Hayley K., and Marika Tiggemann. "Development of Perceived Body Size and Dieting Awareness in Young Girls." *Perceptual and Motor Skills*, vol. 99, no. 3, ser. 1, Dec. 2004, pp. 790–792. *1*, doi:10.2466/pms.99.3.790-792.

Flegal, Katherine M., et al. "Association of All-Cause Mortality With Overweight and Obesity Using Standard Body Mass Index Categories." *Journal of the American Medical Association*, vol. 309, no. 1, 2 Jan. 2013, pp. 71–82., doi:10.1001/jama.2012.113905.

Forney, K. Jean, et al. "The Medical Complications Associated with Purging." *International Journal of Eating Disorders*, vol. 49, no. 3, 2016, pp. 249–259., doi:10.1002/eat.22504.

Fotia, Miranda. "8 Things Everyone Should Know About The Fat Acceptance Movement." *Panda Gossips*, 24 July 2018, pandagossips.com/posts/3123.

Franklin, Joseph C., et al. "Observations on Human Behavior in Experimental Semistarvation and Rehabilitation." *Journal of Clinical Psychology*, vol. 4, no. 1, Jan. 1948, pp. 28–45., doi:10.1002/1097-4679(194801)4:13.0.co;2-f.

Hayes, Sharon, and Stacey Tantleff-Dunn. "Am I Too Fat to Be a Princess? Examining the Effects of Popular Children's Media on Young Girls' Body Image." *British Journal of Developmental Psychology*, vol. 28, no. 2, 23 Dec. 2010, pp. 413–426., doi:10.1348/026151009x424240.

Herskowitz, Amy, and Deb Burgard. *The Problem with Poodle Science.* Performance by Stacy Bias, Association for Size Diversity and Health, 23 Feb. 2015, www.youtube.com/watch?v=H89QQfXtc-k.

International Journal of Yoga (IJoY), Medknow Publications, 2010, www.ijoy.org.in/.

Jordan, Rob. "Stanford Researchers Find Mental Health Prescription: Nature." *Stanford News*, Stanford Woods Institute for the Environment, 9 Apr. 2016, news.stanford.edu/2015/06/30/hiking-mental-health-063015/.

Keys, Ancel, et al. *The Biology of Human Starvation.* Vol. 1-2, University of Minnesota Press, 1950.

Lowes, Jacinta, and Marika Tiggemann. "Body Dissatisfaction, Dieting Awareness and the Impact of Parental Influence in Young Children." *British Journal of Health Psychology*, vol. 8, no. 2, May

2003, pp. 135–147.,
doi:10.1348/135910703321649123.

Mann, Traci. "Why Do Dieters Regain Weight? Calorie
Deprivation Alters Body and Mind, Overwhelming
Willpower." *Psychological Science Agenda* , American
Psychological Association, May 2008,
www.apa.org/science/about/psa/2018/05/calorie-
deprivation.

"Meditation: In Depth." *National Center for Complementary
and Integrative Health*, U.S. Department of Health
and Human Services, Apr. 2016,
nccih.nih.gov/health/meditation/overview.htm.

Ogilvy & Mather Advertising. *Smoking Kid*, Thai Health
Promotion Foundation , 23 June 2012,
www.youtube.com/watch?v=aHrdy6qcumg.

Publishing, Harvard Health. "Sour Mood Getting You
down? Get Back to Nature." *Harvard Health
Publishing*, Harvard Medical School, July 2018,
www.health.harvard.edu/mind-and-mood/sour-
mood-getting-you-down-get-back-to-nature.

"The U.S. Weight Loss & Diet Control Market." *Research
and Markets*, Marketdata LLC, Feb. 2019,
www.researchandmarkets.com/research/qm2gts/the_
72_billion?w=4.

Van der Kolk, Bessel. *The Body Keeps the Score: Brain, Mind,
and Body in the Healing of Trauma*. Penguin Books,
2015.

ACKNOWLEDGMENT TO MY READERS

THANK YOU FOR spending time reading *MeaningFULL*. With such a wide variety of approaches, theories, books, self-help guides, and worksheets that a person might enlist to conquer their food, weight, and body image issues, these pages represent just a portion of what I support personally and professionally. This also means that, with content this broad, there were limitations as to what could be included.

I recognize that powerful experiences related to eating, weight, and body image occur daily. Those can include but are not limited to stigma (e.g., discrimination, "us/them," stereotypes), and healthism (e.g., viewing health as a primary marker of well-being or success). While reading these pages, I hope you felt included and represented. Maybe something resonated in a way that united you with yourself individually or with others communally. Maybe you felt excluded if aspects of your personal story were missing or if something important to you was not mentioned. Respect for our diverse lives and voices is important to me—to all of us. So if you experienced any of the above, I invite you to write about it, talk to a friend, schedule a chat with a professional, blog about it, or write me. *NOTE: Due to ethics and professional limits, I can't and won't respond in the capacity of a therapist but as the author of this book.*

All our voices are important. When we share our experiences respectfully and in safety, we can increase our collective knowledge about and empathy for each other's journeys on the way to conquering our food, weight, and body image issues. I humbly close with this recognition, because we are all connected, and every one of us matters.

ABOUT THE AUTHOR

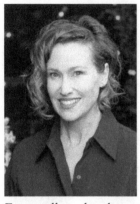 After having dealt with her own 20+ years of eating and body issues ranging from mild frustrations to serious eating disorders, Alli Spotts-De Lazzer became a Licensed Marriage and Family Therapist (#49842) and Licensed Professional Clinical Counselor (#844) specializing in eating and body image issues. Eventually, she became a Certified Eating Disorders Specialist—the only nationally recognized designation indicating a specialty in eating disorders.

Alli has been a featured speaker at public events; presented workshops at national and international conferences, graduate schools, clinical training facilities, and hospitals; published articles in trade magazines, online information hubs, and academic journals; and appeared as an eating disorders expert on local news. She has also co-chaired committees for the International Association of Eating Disorders Professionals (iaedp™) and the Academy for Eating Disorders. In 2017, she received the iaedp™ Member of the Year award.

As far as public activism and advocacy, in 2014, Alli created #ShakeIt for Self-Acceptance!®: a series of public events sparking conversations about body, soul, and self-acceptance through fun, inspiration, and flash mob dance. This movement has appeared across America. Highlights include appearing on Capitol Hill and at the Los Angeles Staples Center. July 13, 2017 was recognized as "#ShakeIt for Self-Acceptance! Day" in the City of Los Angeles by Mayor Eric Garcetti.

Throughout the years, Alli has witnessed firsthand that stories of humanness, joy, inspiration, and hope increase people's receptivity to both considering change and opening up to education. That motivated her to create *MeaningFULL*.

ABOUT THE PRESS

Unsolicited Press was founded in 2012 and is based in Portland, Oregon. The small press publishes fiction, poetry, and creative nonfiction written by award-winning and emerging authors.

Learn more at www.unsolicitedpress.com

CPSIA information can be obtained
at www.ICGtesting.com
Printed in the USA
BVHW031934250121
598700BV00009B/252

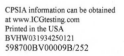